I HAVE BEEN TALKING WITH YOUR DOCTOR:

FIFTY DOCTORS TALK ABOUT THE HEALTHCARE CRISIS
AND THE DOCTOR-PATIENT RELATIONSHIP

BY PEGGY A. ROTHBAUM, PH. D.

I HAVE BEEN TALKING WITH YOUR DOCTOR:

FIFTY DOCTORS TALK ABOUT THE HEALTHCARE CRISIS
AND THE DOCTOR-PATIENT RELATIONSHIP

BY PEGGY A. ROTHBAUM, PH.D.

ISBN 978-0-9883592-9-1

PEGGY A. ROTHBAUM, PH.D.
doctorprothbaum@gmail.com
http://www.drpeggyrothbaum.com

232 SAINT PAUL STREET
WESTFIELD, NJ 07090

CONTENTS

Dedication

I dedicate this book:

To my own doctors, out of incredible gratitude to them for taking such good care of me. I don't know where I would be without them.

To my doctor interviewees, with utmost respect for them and with outrage and frustration at the way that they are treated with such disrespect.

To the public and our legislators, in the hope that this book will help them to understand and take action about the disturbing state of the healthcare crisis.

To patients everywhere. *We need our doctors.*

FOREWORD

I am pleased to have been asked to write the Foreword for this wonderful book. Dr. Peggy Rothbaum has thoughtfully encapsulated one of the most serious social and political issues that we face as nation today: Why is the doctor patient-relationship eroding and how does this impact our health and well being?

Rather than writing lengthy paragraphs on her personal views, she has gone to a primary source of medical care, collecting extremely candid and moving experiences by individually interviewing 50 physicians, spanning many subspecialties, from primary care to neurosurgery.

Using their own words, Dr. Rothbaum uncovers the significant source of anguish that our medical system imposes on both patients and doctors alike. As an expert and published author in conflict resolution and health policy, she defines the problem and explores potential solutions.

Rather than shying away from the dissatisfaction that we feel and deeming the problem too complex to tackle, her work displays an honesty and dedication to the art and science of medical healing. By listening to doctors tell their own concerns, which are consistent across gender of clinician, years in practice, and whether he or she is in primary care or subspecialty practice, she reveals the depth of this troubling issue.

Dr. Rothbaum has been in practice as a psychologist, collaborating with physicians, for over 25 years. Prior to starting her practice, she earned research credentials in educational statistics and measurement and completed a post-doctoral fellowship in mental health research. She has over 50 publications, most of which address healthcare concerns. Dr. Rothbaum has also served as a contributor to healthcare Op-Ed publications in New Jersey's Star Ledger, The Record, and Courier News, as well as The Daily Oklahoman. She has been a contributor to the national publication, Medical Economics. Dr. Rothbaum has served on numerous advisory boards serving diverse patient populations, spanning cancer survivors to children with developmental disabilities. She draws from this broad professional experience to ask questions that provided a portal to the circumspect answers from our health care community.

Dr. Rothbaum's insightful, albeit disturbing, book offers us an opportunity to take a serious warning, a step back, and to ask ourselves, as we age, will we be happy with who is taking care of us, or will we be harkening back to a golden age of medicine, like a Renaissance statue that will never be replicated?

Claire Boccia Liang, M.D., FACC
Director, Women's Heart Program
Morristown Medical Center
Atlantic Health System, Morristown, New Jersey

INTRODUCTION

WHY I AM WRITING THE BLOG AND THE BOOK, I HAVE BEEN TALKING WITH YOUR DOCTOR.

It is for three reasons:

1. Out of incredible gratitude to my own doctors

2. With utmost respect for my doctor colleagues and with outrage and frustration at the way they are treated with such disrespect

3. To educate the public and our legislators about the disturbing state of the healthcare crisis

SAMPLE AND METHODOLOGY

I interviewed 50 doctors using about 4 pages of questions that I developed based on the professional research literature on doctoring and my personal professional experience working with doctors.

My request at the beginning of each interview was: With the exception of the first few questions which are demographics (such as specific educational degrees and years in practice post-residency), which I would like to have answered, answer those questions that you wish to answer, skip the ones that you wish to skip. They get repetitive towards the end, as you will see. I want to get as much information as possible. I have also had a few interviewees tell me that they want to talk about something else, which is fine. It ends up being the same information anyway.

I started the process by interviewing my own doctors and colleagues. The interviews lasted between 30 minutes and two hours, depending on how much time each doctor had and if they wanted to talk longer. Most of them were about an hour long. After each interview I asked each interviewee if they could refer me to a colleague who might be interested in being interviewed. So, I ended up interviewing doctors who I had not known previously. I made contact with a letter and phone calls, using the name of the doctor who had referred me. After they agreed to be interviewed, I went to their offices one by one. They talked, I typed. They met with me in between patients, taking breaks to answer emails, texts, phone calls, or deal with emergencies, or after hours, on time off, during paperwork time, or while eating a rushed meal.

After completing the interviews, I am left with an even deeper understanding of the health care crisis. In addition to being in practice as a psychologist, I am a researcher and health care policy analyst. I stay informed about the crisis... or, so I thought. However, it is worse than I ever imagined. The insurance companies are dictating rationed, inadequate, insufficient health care for most of us. This leaves the doctors who I interviewed, as well as their colleagues, in a totally untenable situation which they juggle and manage with skill, compassion and dedication that is beyond impressive. It is my hope that these interviews will expose an intimate portrait of the gravity and urgency of our healthcare crisis. It is with the utmost gratitude, admiration and humility that I thank my doctor interviewees for their help with this task.

CHAPTER 1

DEMOGRAPHICS OF THE DOCTOR INTERVIEWEES

GENDER

Male	32
Female	18

PRIMARY CARE/SPECIALISTS

Primary Care	25
Specialists	25

AGE OF PATIENTS

Children and adolescents only	8
Adults only	23
Both	19

SPECIALIST TYPE	
Cardiology	OBGYN
Endocrinology	Ophthalmology
Gastroenterology	Orthopedics
Infectious diseases	Plastic surgery
Immunology	Rheumatology
Nephrology	Urology
Neurosurgery	

YEARS IN PRACTICE	
Years	# of Doctors
<5	0
6–10	6
11–15	2
16–20	10
21–25	9
26–30	10
31–35	5
36–40	4
41–45	2
46–50	1
51–55	1
TOTAL	50
Full or partially retired	4

CHAPTER 2

BEING A DOCTOR

Introduction and rationale for this book

* There is a lot of published literature on the experience
  of being a doctor. I have read much of it over the years
  and I went back to it before conducting the interviews
  for my book. The vast majority of this literature
  discusses the rewards for doctors of taking care of
  patients.This also includes topics such as doctor-
  patient communication, how to choose a doctor,
  understanding medications, coping with office visits,
  improving health habits, and coping with physical
  and psychological symptoms of post-traumatic stress
  disorder (PTSD). The rationale of my doctor book is
  not much different than these books. The problem is
  that healthcare has deteriorated so dramatically in the
  years since these books were written. And there is so
  much damage to the doctor-patient relationship. These
  new developments, and how they have changed the
  experience of being a doctor, are not mentioned in the
  books that I have read over the years.

I also read some of the books where doctors tell how
they feel about being doctors. Some of them are about
juggling the grueling clinical hours involved with class
work, learning to interact with patients — and the long
schedules of being "on call" — with compassion for
patients and one's own feelings. As someone who has
physician friends and colleagues, I will tell you that it
is hard to comprehend the difficulty of their schedules.
Again, this situation has become worse in the intervening

years since these books were written. I know, because I asked my doctor interviewees to tell me about it.

The books by medical students and resident physicians caught my attention when I was a graduate student. Graduate school was difficult for me. It was a lot of hours, typically multiple simultaneous jobs, and financial stress, all of which imposed on my personal life. But the schedules of a medical student or resident physician were a whole different matter. The people who lived across the hall were medical students and residents when I was in graduate school. Their schedules were insane. I graduated with what seemed to me to be a lot of debt, but they graduated with several hundred thousand dollars of debt. My work was important. Mental health is related to everything that matters. But it seemed to me that their work had a pressure and urgency that my work did not have as part of it. Literally, their work was life and death. In addition to having serious doubts that I could even pass organic chemistry, allegedly the "make or break" course to get accepted to medical school, I was pretty sure that I could not handle the intense and unrelenting pressure that they had to manage every day.

Those of us who went to college remember the pre-med students. They were the ones who studied all the time. There was tremendous pressure to excel. They took multiple difficult science courses at the same time, some of which were "make or break" if they did not get an A. They were always in the library. They had a lot of labs and lab reports. They all seemed very smart, and much smarter than me. As one of my interviewees summarized the situation, "Most people aren't committed at such a young age at everything. My kids aren't either. I was so focused in high school. You have to want to be a physician early on. You have to focus early on or you are already way behind the eight ball. You have to have the dedication and the commitment. The kids in their 20s, they are partying at night. The people in medical school can't do that. We had tests. We were sitting in the library or on call. Studying and studying."

So, why do it? Why become a doctor?

Q: WHY DID YOU BECOME A DOCTOR?

* My doctor interviewees told me about it. Their commitment to helping people is palpable. Some doctors also looked for a way to combine science with interacting with people. There was clinical fascination with medicine and curiosity about the complexities of the human body. There was frequently the influence or wanting to be like a family member who was a doctor. Personal tragedy was often motivating factor. Some wanted to be a doctor as children; some discovered their interest along the way. One interviewee summarized it as, "I was good at science. I wanted to work with people and make a difference. Few fields combine the two."

- *Obviously to help people. Growing up I was deathly afraid of blood, everything that was gross, and the body. One day I transcended that and thought that I could make a difference.*

- *The only thing I wanted to be at 5.*

- *It was a complex combination of wanting to be in a meaningful profession and helping people. I wanted to be in a profession where I didn't have to wonder when I went home at night if my time was well spent.*

- *From a young age, I found it fascinating and it was* always *my desire.*

- *To help people. A family member died of cancer when I was a child. I couldn't understand why they couldn't just take out the cancer.*

- *I was good at science. I wanted to work with people and make a difference. Few fields combine the two.*

- *I like to solve medical puzzles.*

- *Having a sick father. He died young.*

- *I like science and I like people.*

- *A close relative was very sick and I was very involved.*

- *I went into my subspecialty to take care of families in a long term way and help them take care of their disease over the long term and have a relationship with them.*

- *I want to be a doctor since 4. I had a sick cousin who died as a teenager when I was 5. I don't remember a time when I wasn't going to be a doctor.*

- *Because I felt that I wanted to work in an area where I was developing skills and an ability, where getting older would mean getting wiser and more skillful. And I wanted to work with people.*

- *Drawn to science. Originally I was a biomedical engineer, but the softer science of dealing with people drew me in.*

- *I had an uncle who was a surgeon and who was my inspiration. He encouraged me.*

- *I just love people and I wanted to help them and be near them and make a difference.*

- *Something I always wanted to do. Never saw myself doing anything else.*

- *I wanted to be a doctor like my old time pediatrician.*

- *I like science and I like interacting with people.*

- *I wanted to help people, being selfless and offering my skills to people to make them feel better, like my father.*

- *To heal people.*

* In a related question, I asked:

Q: What are the most desirable qualities of a doctor? What are the necessary skills and abilities?

* Similar to the reasons why they became a doctor, the responses from the doctor interviewees to this question were a mix of the need for both caring and clinical skills. Clinical skills included basic intelligence, a fund of scientific knowledge, curiosity, the ability and willingness to tackle and resolve complex problems, to juggle a lot of facts simultaneously, The caring skills mentioned included empathy, patience, sensitivity to individual differences, compassion, humility, and of course the ability to listen and communicate. I wanted to separate these responses into those two categories for easier reading, but I was able to do it. They are so intertwined. Medicine, it seems, is as much of an art as it is a science. "It's a given that you know the medicine and the science very well", said one doctor interviewee, but as another one said, "You have to care."

* Caring, and being able to show it, was mentioned by all interviewees.

- *Good listener. Most people don't even need a good answer, if someone just listened.*

- *Personality. You have to touch your patients both physically and emotionally. My father had a quote on his desk which I used as my high school year book quote. "What is that imaginative gift that some people have of making others feel competent, important and esteemed." This is necessary for a physician.*

- *Obviously, to realize that you are a servant and that you need to prepare yourself in the best possible way to serve your patients. You need to listen to your patients attentively and with compassion.*

* Most doctor interviewees also mentioned the importance of caring combined with clinical skills.

- *Compassion, intelligence, interest in the field, learning from patients.*

- *Smart and compassionate is equally important. Have to have the ability to talk to all kinds of people. I have had good experience with people. Some people come to me with mistrust of other doctors and I build trust.*

- *Above average intelligence. You need to be able to think outside the box to some degree. And it would be helpful if you have a good disposition so that you can interact positively with your patients.*

- *Twofold. You have your scientific qualities and the ability to keep up with the proper medicine and proper testing to be ordered and staying up to date that occur and a moving science. On the other hand you have communication skills and the ability to try and treat the patient as best you can base on situation. Some of the specialists are good at what they do but have trouble communicating or their patients don't like them, it's one problem you can sit and talk with me. In a perfect world you have both things going on.*

- *To be compassionate, humble, a good listener, and have good ability for science and clinical skills.*

- *Intelligence and skill and above all, compassion. You can love them to death but you have to fix them. Have to have ethics and compassion. Manual dexterity and vision. Have to have some insight into people and how their minds work, how they describe complaints and how you put together how they think. Relate to patients as people.*

- *Intelligent and inquisitive and have a mind that can do deductive medical thinking. Have the empathic communication skills that are necessary to elicit information that you need. You can be brilliant but if they are pissed off at how you ask the questions or you don't understand you will not get their mind. Like a detective and thinking outside the box. The compassion and human skills to bring it all together with communication skills.*

- *Good listener. Have to be interested in the body and fascinated by it. Have to have a calling. Empathy. Curiosity. A smile has to be there.*

- *Concern for sick, ill people. Compassion, physical skills, understanding.*

- *Good listener. Open, non-judgmental. Disciplined in skills. Up to date.*

- *Good listener. Good detective. Good communicator.*

- *I would say it's the combination of merging high tech and high touch. You need a knowledge base. You need to know stuff or where to get it. Medical resources are getting better. You need to have that. And you need to be a mensch. You need to teach people to fish.*

- *Compassion and being able to put oneself in the other's shoes. Have to be analytical and not mentally lazy and thorough. And you have to put the patient first. Other specialties need a different skill set, I am a primary care doctor.*

- *Communication, which mostly involves listening. It's a given that you know the medicine and the science very well.*

- *You have to be knowledgeable. Inquisitive, compassionate.*

- *A large fund of knowledge and be able to connect with people on a personal level well. To be a clinical and personal education so that people feel cared for by me. The holy grail is so hard to achieve, is an adequate fund of knowledge, clinical acumen and diagnostic acumen along with a bedside manner and combining all of this. Can have all of the book knowledge, but if you can't make your patient open up, you could miss what is wrong. All three of these is what I am striving for.*

- *The ability to listen and take history. To do analysis via history taking.*

- *Good communication skills, patience, sense of humor*

- *To have empathy, compassion, and excellent use of the knowledge that they have acquired. To be able to properly diagnose and treat illnesses.*

- *You have to listen to what the person is telling you and what they are not telling you. You have to be completely open when you walk in the door. It's not what it says on the sheet even if the person thinks that it is. Care for them like a family member. The medicine is not that hard. It's perseverance and dedication that gets you through school. Anyone could figure out the material. You have to care.*

- * Other doctor interviewees talked about juggling the demanding requirements of being a doctor.

- *Good communication skills, being intelligent, having a good memory and knowing how to use your computer. The ability to juggle.*

- *Empathy. We all get jaded at some level, but you have to be empathetic towards what the patient is feeling. Sort through* massive amounts of information and drill down to what is necessary. Have to go without sleep. A lot of my patients could not do this job. They want out of work notes. Most are wonderful. But they don't really know what it takes to do this job.

• You have to follow up. Can't say it's Saturday and I am not on call, or I will look at it tomorrow. You have to take care of it now. You have to be nice to people. Treat patients like families.

* Persistence and not giving up are also important requirements.

• Humanism, skills and abilities that depend on the type of medicine. To know what you don't know and when you need to ask.

• You have to be a perfectionist. You have to want to continually learn and learn from patients. You have to be technically skilled. You have to filter material and accumulate a knowledge base for your own algorithm to diagnose. You have to be extremely ethical. You have to be professional.

• This is hard. The humanistic qualities. You have to really care about people on a very personal level. Have to be able to listen. Have to have good observational skills. What someone is saying is not what their body is telling you. Have to be stubborn and work hard, have persistence and some intelligence. Some OCD. Make sure things add up and you have checked every box that you have to check.

• Dedication. And diligence. I would rather have a doctor who cares if I get better than one at the top of the field. People vary in skills. Have to have a desire to want to continue to learn.

* Some of the interviewees also talked about the need to recognize limits in their own abilities, in addition to caring in order to be good being a doctor.

- *Empathy. Good listening skills. Knowing what you don't know. Having a sixth sense.*

- *Other than obviously intelligence and understanding: compassion. Having a heart and listening and using the five senses when dealing with a patient. That is almost more important than actual medical knowledge. It is the key. Know a lot about a little and being able to know what you know and know when to refer.*

- *You have to have an adequate fund of information and knowledge and be sensitive to needs of patients. And care for the patients and have some degree of personal interest in their patients. Have to be able to continue to learn and explore the new corridors of medicine. A little bit humbling in this day and age. We get the sh.t beat out of us by everyone and can't take it personally.*

- *Education. Compassion, humility and sympathy for patients. Skills and abilities come with training and with time but you have to develop a bonding with the patient. The doctor patient is a relationship it's not just business.*

- *Caring. Being compassionate and empathetic. More important than having knowledge and being super smart. Can have the worst bedside manner and be concerned about things that are causing them more stress than the disease, ie family and finances. You have to put yourself in their shoes, which brings the art of medicine in to play rather than being book smart and acting like you know everything. Obviously, you have to have education and be good at your specialty. It varies among physicians. Ability to cope with lot of sick people and move onto the next patient you can help and realize you can't help everyone. Have limits like everything else. Medicine has its limits. You learn that along the way more so as you get older.*

• *Empathy is huge. I am pretty good at that. You have to have patience. My brother says I have built in Prozac. Check your ego at the door to be a good doctor. My knowledge is broad but not deep. Know your limits and when you need to consult.*

* Flexibility to adapt to change is necessary.

• *Having the clinical ability to integrate and learn the material. Plus all of the humanistic things. Empathy. Ability to listen and communicate. And knowing what to do and doing it. Today multitasking and to deal with a high level of stress and not project it onto others, managerial and financial skills and computer skills. It has changed.*

• *Caring, sensitivity and the ability to hear and understand each patient as an individual. Focus and pay attention and listen to what the patient is trying to tell you. You have to care enough about the patient to understand background history, like social and family history and their impact on emotional and medical well being.*

• *Compassion and empathy, wisdom to be able to accurately make the diagnosis and to anticipate complications and to be able to take care of the whole person not just physically, but mentally. To be a very good communicator in the language of the person you are dealing with. To be able to interact with peers and other people in the medical profession and to be able to include them in your practice and approach to the patient. To work with nurses and ancillary services. To be able to quickly arrive at the right conclusions regarding diagnoses. To be able to understand the patients' background and work with the limitations that they give.*

- *It is essential to be able to synthesize disparate pieces of information and to have a mental framework to piece seeming unrelated bits of information into a cohesive story. Plenty of patience and empathy and most importantly to have an open mind. If you look at the patients in front of you through a prism of their disease or appearance etc you won't be able to follow or process the story that they are telling you. People come in all sorts of shapes and sizes with all sorts of unexpected traumas. They all want to be listened to and taken care of with dignity and respect.*

- *Intelligence, empathy, manual dexterity, good observer and listener. Flexible and have an open mind. Have to be able to deal with change. Change in the rules of how healthcare is delivered and in societal values and mores. You have to take care of your own physical health and mental outlook.*

* One doctor mentioned how what it takes to be a good doctor has changed for the worse. Being flexible is not enough.

- *The qualities that a doctor needs in 2015 are different than in the 80s. In the 80s it was to be sympathetic, intelligent and always take care of the patient first. In 2015, you have to watch the bottom line or you get kicked off of the insurance panels and the hospitals and cannot earn a living. It is not most important to take care of people.*

Q: PLEASE TELL ME ABOUT A TYPICAL DAY OR WEEK FOR YOU.

* These responses were not surprising to me, because as I mentioned previously, I had seen it with my across the hall neighbors in graduate school. It doesn't end with residency. The intensity continues throughout the doctors' careers.

• *I average 60 hours a week plus the on call. On call is evenings taking calls from patients. Weekends and holidays taking calls and going to the hospital to see the patients in the hospitals.*

• *I gave up going to the hospital. I used to spend a lot of time there. I got up at 4:30 and came here at 8:30. The money paid for going to the hospital is not worth it. But I feel badly about the lack of continuity of care. I get here at the office at 8:30 and see patients until 4:30 or 5. I see 25-28 people a day. That's not bad. Some people see 50. I don't see how they can do it. Shameful. Our phones never stop. The pre-authorization and insurance bullshit never stops.*

• *Wake up at 5:30 or 6. Go to hospital and make rounds. Do grand rounds and see patients in the office. Do chores. Make phone calls: messages, lab results, family calls, other doctor calls. And then back to the hospital to make rounds.*

• *Pretty chaotic. I mix seeing patients and management, but it doesn't get compartmentalized. One flows into the other and vice versa. I do report and phone calls when I am home at night. Lots of multi tasking. Lots of interruptions. The best times are when I am alone with the patient. I get a lot of gratification out of that. That is the doctoring part. The hardest part of doctoring is time management and the administrative work not related to the patient: Record keeping and other things.*

- *Getting up around 4:30. If I have a real pressing amount of administrative work, I do that first. I try to go to the gym for half an hour. Then go to work by 7:15. If I have too much work and I was too tired the night before, I might work for an hour. In the day there is barely a bathroom break. At 8:15 I might go and see two or three hospitalized patients before 9am office hours start. I usually see patients through my lunch hour. First bathroom break is around 12:30. Microwave food and eat until 12:45, making calls all through. From 1-5, I am seeing patients and dealing with patient issues. Maybe until 5:30. Once the last patients are finished I might have tests that take time to interpret, or make calls, or I might see more patients. I typically don't get home until 7:30. I see my kids for an hour or an hour and a half until they have to hit the sack at 8:30. Usually by 9:30 I am exhausted and I drag myself upstairs to bed fall asleep on the couch. Maybe by 10. I have call weekends every fourth weekend. This is 6am -2pm nonstop in the hospital or 8pm depending what is going on in the hospital. Usually at least a solid six or eight hours a day. I try and do it earlier and earlier in the day so that I have more time with the children. This is for the whole weekend.*

- *It's 24/7.*

- *I still see my own hospitalized patients. I am at the hospital 6:30. Office at 8. I start seeing patients at 8 or 8:30. Take an hour for lunch. Eat breakfast and lunch at my desk. See patients until 4:30 or 5. Leave the office at 7. Have dinner. Often 30-60 more minutes of work at home. That is my day. I see patients for half the day on Friday. I catch up on Friday afternoon. I can usually get to the Y. I see patients at 1 on Thursdays so I can sleep an hour later. I typically put too much in on that morning though.*

- *Get up at 5:15. Go to the hospital or nursing home and do rounds. Office hours and go back to the nursing home. Work 'til 7 or 8. If my kids have something to do or I want to be there, I break and then go back. I am on call 24/7. Always on.*

- *I have always been in a group practice. The days you work, you work very hard, but you have your days off. Before electronics, if you were off, you are off. Partners would take care of it. I work 10 hour days, seven or eight hours seeing patients, then following up on results, messages and doing paperwork. I average four days a week. I don't mind always being connected. I used to come home to a big pile of messages and charts. At the end of the day now I take out my iPad and knock off 20-30 messages. My spouse is asleep and kids are asleep. I can send a message if something needs to be handled. I take my iPad with me where ever I go.*

- *All different. Monday I go to nursing homes to do consults. Today I did two consults. I did follow ups on five other people. These people are pretty sick. One had already gone back to the hospital before I even got the labs back. Then I went to the hospital and did consults and followed up patients. Got here to the office around 12:30 then stayed until 6 and did paperwork. Went home and got dinner going.*

- *I am usually up between 5:30 and 6. I go to the hospital and make rounds on my patients. Then I come to the office. On certain days I also go to nursing homes and see patients there. That varies on the day.*

- *Try for a mix between family and work. But we work seven days a week. By and large we live a nice lifestyle, but we are always working. Never have 24 hours off. We get 2am phone calls on a regular basis. Rarely that both of us sleep all night. I moonlight and do part time work. I have the nanny there because we might both be out at 2am. I often miss family* events. In Disney World I was taking calls. Skiing in Vail, taking phone calls. We don't go anywhere without two cars. I can't have a beat up car. I have to get there. If I am late someone could die or have a different outcome for the rest of their life. In a corporate world, being late 15 minutes is nothing.

- Pretty hectic. Now I have a partner and it is a lot better. I go to one or two hospitals before coming to the office and see 15-25 patients before getting to the office. Then in the office I see 10-15. I get a million calls, texts, and a lot of forms to fill out.

Q: WHAT ARE YOUR GREATEST STRENGTHS AS A DOCTOR?

* Interestingly, when the doctors answered this question, their focus was mostly on the caring aspects of doctoring, not the clinical or scientific aspects.

- My ability to reassure a patient and take time; my empathy.

- I am passionate about what I do in both my professional and personal life. This has proven to be one of my greatest strengths. I hold hands and I cry with my patients.

- I think that I am a good listener. That is very important. I can tell when patients are trying to tell me indirectly, which comes with time and experience. Giving strength to people doesn't always come from medicine. Being supportive and understanding and listening. Sometimes patient know there is no cure and they will not get better and don't want to hear it. In that case everything you do for them is appreciated and doesn't take rocket science to fix it.

- I like to think that it makes it easier to do my job if I just put myself in the same position as my patients. I picture them as my family members if I am at the doctor myself. It becomes not about me. It's more about them and it helps me practice *consistently. I genuinely like to talk to people, although it can be a lot harder if I am an hour behind. Sometimes I am getting behind because I have been talking with someone for 20 minutes. A nice thing about medicine is I feel like I am off a treadmill.*

- *My empathy.*
- *Empathy.*
- *My ability to listen to people and to see them as a member of my family.*
- *Mine is my personality and my communication and connection with patients is at a high level. And I am pretty smart. I am a great doctor after 30 years in. I have reached a lot of the places where I want my trainees to go.*
- *I think that the reason that I am so busy here is that I grew up here. Middle class blue collar area. It's how I grew up. My dad was a dock worker. I can relate to my patients pretty well.*
- *Listening. And personality wise, I am down to earth. I get along with my patients like friends.*
- *Relationships and communication.*
- *Listen to the patient. To think is the most important skill. People know more book knowledge than I do but they do not think.*
- *A gestalt for illness. The ability to make the patients feel my compassion.*
- *I think that I am able to relate to my patients.*
- *On parallel with my weaknesses as a business man-doctor. I enjoy spending time talking with people. I have never had a volume type of practice. So many doctors have come to the conclusion that you have to make a choice: Run a business*

or take care of business. These two things are not compatible. I have made the financially unwise but professionally more rewarding choice to practice this way.

- *I am very much a people person. Look people in the eye when you speak to them. Allow the patient to feel as comfortable as they want with you. Some doctors don't want contact. I have gone to parties, funeral, and baptisms. I try to make an appearance even if it's 15 minutes. My patients know how much I care about them. Empathize or sympathize. If a patient stops seeing me, I want to know why. If it's financial I will do almost everything legal to make it work. It bothers me.*

- *Being present and letting patients know that I have time for them no matter how small the problem seems to them. If it is the only visit that day that is normal, it's great for both of us. A patient said, "I like coming here because no matter how small my problem is, I know that you will treat it with respect."*

- *I am a pretty good listener and have a pretty good sixth sense that keeps me out of trouble.*

- *I can connect with people. This helps them to get out their medical problems.*

* Persistence and not giving up are mentioned again as crucial skills.

- *Compassion and listening to patients and knowing what you don't know. I told the residents and interns, you see 40-50 patients day. Only one or two will really need your help. The rest will get better just by seeing you. Do no good and do no harm. This belies all of the mandates like the EMR, the pay for performance, exams, all of the caps all of the licenses. Your major role is evaluation and to determine if the condition is self limiting. Today we have the quest for the diagnosis and this promotes the cost of medical care. In 90% of the time you don't need a diagnosis because the condition is self-limiting.*

- *My patience. The patients are so needy and I sit and listen and try and help them. This is also why I run late. I sit and let them take their time to say it. Am I the smartest? No. But I am smart about knowing when to ask. The computer is a friend. I knew it once, I can look it up.*

- *My desire to help people and seek out new information, new techniques, and new technology.*

- *I am dogged. I will research things. I will spend time finding what is the most likely diagnosis. I am compulsive. I communicate well with the patients. I call them back and call them to check on them out of the blue.*

- *I care and I listen. I know when I don't know the answer and I know where to find it.*

- *Ability to diagnose by listening to the patient. Understanding lab work and physical examinations and using them to prescribe or refer appropriately if beyond general pediatrics skills and abilities to subspecialist.*

- *Endurance. Handling unpredictable hours and unscheduled crises.*

- *I always do what I have chosen to do. I listen and I don't give up. I work on the problem until I get a solution. Typically my patients have reached dead ends with other physicians.*

- *I think about what the patient is telling me, analyze, try to figure out the answer. Try to make it fit into a diagnosis.*

* Clinical skills, of course, are important.

• *Interest. I enjoy the work.*

• *Skills and ability. Compassion and compulsiveness. I tell students not to go into it if they don't have that. Something noble about helping a fellow human being. I feel better giving physical and emotional support. I get satisfaction. I'm not very smart but I make up for it in other ways.*

• *Empathy. Compassion. Patience. I am pretty good problem solver and listener. Patients say that they are comfortable and can tell me anything.*

• *I am intelligent. Not the smartest, but I am intelligent. I have good manual dexterity and an ability to envision things and what could be there, not just now. I can imagine things differently. I come from a non-medical family and this is a huge strength. I have to explain to my family. My parents were in sales and customer relations. I can perceive what is going on, not just what they are saying. What is actually going on. What is not being said as well as what is being said.*

• *Good communicator. Good diagnostician.*

• *My ability to reason, solve problems, observe and listen and care.*

• *I am pretty good at communicating with patients and listening and working together. I know what I am doing. I administer this practice. I deal with it.*

• *I am a good listener. I really enjoy getting the information that I get to need for doing the right thing for the family. I like to look and I like that process. I really care about everything.*

• *My caring. Knowing what I don't know. I care about my patients' health. I have a good memory. I am kind of funny. I am good at multitasking.*

- *I have to toot my own horn? I think that I am able to encompass all of the different aspects of medicine when I approach a patient and I am able to deal with it. My peers like me and people who deal with me enjoy working with me. My patients feel that I am very compassionate and empathic towards them I am told that I talk to them in a way that they understand. I am able to find solutions to problems that other people miss.*

- *Ability to listen. Deductive reasoning.*

- *I can't answer. I believe that I am well regarded though because I care about my patients and put in a lot of time with them. And I am experienced.*

Q: What was your greatest joy in your career as a doctor

* Again, many times the responses of the doctor interviewees were from their hearts: a caring response about the importance of their interactions with their patients.

- *The interaction with the patients.*

- *One of my patients told me to tell my mother thank you for giving birth to me.*

- *I really get a lot of joy when I hear from people, not directly from them, I hear through someone else. "He's really great to talk to," or "He's great with kids." It makes me feel good.*

- *I know it sounds stupid but I get such joy when patients thank me. So many people are so nasty and entitled. And when they thank me… One patient's son thanked me and said, "This visit was worth its weight in gold."*

- *I can't think of one greatest joy. I like teaching. I like when students are with me. Being able to be there for a patient and getting the appreciation from the patient.*

- *Saving patients who would be dying or near death.*

- *Years with families. Best times and worst times. Babies grown up and having babies in long-term connections. I was a support person to talk to about the worst times and anxieties. I can calm people down from a bad place to a softer place. I don't save lives. But I also watch trainees when they grow up and see them doing things that I taught them.*

- *Watching children grow up. Patients grew up and became parents — I took care of a second generation and one case of third generation. Went to a wedding. At the pre-ceremony I spoke briefly. I knew him and his father. Bumping into people who remember that I was their pediatrician.*

- *A sense of engaging with people who otherwise would be abandoned. We are fix-it people. We don't dwell on the negative.*

- *Delivering a baby. I delivered several.*

- *Not one. When things go well for a patient who wasn't doing well. I do procedures and they can look like they are going to die and maybe 15 minutes later look okay. The patients and their loved ones are grateful and have become loyal patients. Those are often the proudest moments.*

- *Having the privilege to do it.*

- *I don't have one. When I find something that nobody else found, or making a patient feel better. Today a patient said she has always been afraid of doctors but she will come back and see me.*

- *Relationships*

- *I can't think of one. Every week there is something that gives me a high. For example: I ask patients if they are gay, straight, bi, or undecided. One woman started to cry. She had never been able to tell her doctor. It was over then. Every week there is something that recommits me to this and reminds me why I am here.*

- *I have so many. My greatest joy is to be able to impact for example couples who were about to divorce, restructure their lives and avoid divorce. To witness or to assist a baby being born who at the beginning of the pregnancy was under tremendous risk of being aborted.*

- *There are a lot. Not a single one. It feels good when people appreciate you and what you have done. And knowing that you are making a huge difference. I have saved a lot of lives. They don't all appreciate it, but the ones who do really do.*

- *Really making a difference in a child's life. When I know because of my skills and education and training I have been able to save a child's life and keep that family intact.*

- *To find people healed and to enable them to live a normal life.*

- *When people say I feel well cared for. I feel like I can handle that problem. Someone walking out the door feeling better when they leave. The healing aspect.*

- *I can't pick out an individual thing that I did. The greatest thing is when a patient comes in three or four years later and says doc you did this and this and it changed my life. Most of the time I can't remember what I did, but it is nice validation that I have an impact on patients.*

- *Telling people that they are healthy.*

- *Helping people. Seeing patient do well even though they had complicated problems.*

- *When you see improvement in a patient or who turns around and the prevention of suffering.*

- *It is when I really get to have time and look at someone in their eyes and understand something about them that I may not have understood before and figure out how they tick. It may just be to see the relief that washes over them. I cannot cure everyone but there is a lot of relief that I can give someone. The Latin root of doctor has nothing to do with healing, it means teacher. I cannot tell you how to live or be, but can tell you a better choice. I speak medicine and you speak patient so that our job is to translate it into English so that we can both understand. I try to choose what I know about the patients' work or household terms so that the patient can understand.*

* There is also pride in clinical accomplishments.
- *Just making it through graduating medical school after a long school career. Finally getting out. Then you realize it is not always better; sometimes miss those days. It's interesting. Best joy is helping people. Make their last few years as enjoyable as possible.*
- *Graduation. Starting practice. Having one of my sons enter medicine.*
- *I graduated summa cum laude from medical school.*
- *Getting into my particular subspecialty and taking my boards.*
- *I don't know if I have one. I don't have extremes. My first one was taking care of an elbow. I clicked it back in.*
- *I cannot pick one. If you make a difficult diagnosis and you really can help someone. My best day is when someone comes and thanks me. Thank you for helping me or finding this or whatever. For example, in the case of an obscure diagnosis.*
- *Being independently employed.*

- *Having created an organization that delivers health care in a superior way for the benefit of the staff and the patients.*

- *Ability to listen and think.*

- *Doing the right things.*

- *When somebody does really well. When people do well who are not expected to do well. Medicine has improved and we can help with a lot of things that we used to not be able to help. With supportive and preventive care this does not happen the same way. Medicine has improved so much. This gives me great joy that we can help people a lot now.*

- *One of the main things is being involved in teaching the new generation of doctors to try and emphasize in my way what I think are important qualities of being a doctor. By modeling compassion, empathy, dedication, follow-through professionalism advocacy. A real privilege to help train other physicians. This career pathway because I was so impressed with the doctors who mentored me in residency and training. I couldn't think of anyone I would rather emulate. A good way to honor my mentors by trying to pass on the key positive things that they taught me to the next generation. Creates some new stresses, but alleviates some stress — satisfaction from doing it.*

Misc
- *I don't know.*

- *Too numerous to count.*

Q: What was your proudest moment as a doctor?

* Again, there is the consistent emphasis on the caring aspects of being a doctor.

- *Helping people who never thought that they would ever been able to get better, get better.*

- *A family member almost died in a car crash. I helped to save his life. I learned that I have an intuitive ability. He almost died. But he didn't. It transformed our relationship in an odd way. That was a proud and joyful moment and a rite of passage and the beginnings of healings. It became important to do this for friends and family.*

- *People feel like they can, some, rely on me for support and they have confidence in my ability. I know that I make their lives better.*

- *Moments. Giving family members peace at the time of their loved one's death. Great reward for a job well done.*

- *Always those cases in the ICU who are sick and thought to be dead and sometimes can bring them back and they get discharged from the hospital. Being recognized in the community as trustworthy and colleagues send me patients they don't feel comfortable handling or they call me in the middle of the night for my opinion.*

* Of course, there is pride in clinical accomplishments.

- *Awards and recognition by school, staff of hospital and students for me.*

- *The day I graduated from med school I saw my dad crying for the first time. He wanted to be a doctor and his parents didn't have the money to support him to be a doctor*

- *When I became a fellow of the Academy of Physicians at a very young age.*

- *Practicing with two family members.*

- *Being on health advisory panel for the State of New Jersey and I was able to implement low risk procedures in hospitals that didn't have them. I was able to open up these programs in community hospitals.*

- *I was raised that pride is a bad thing. But I am proud when I have a really successful surgery.*

- *Being on a plane delivering a baby and getting a thank you. Becoming president of my state society and being named physician of the year and getting the founders day award from two schools the same.*

- *Not one. I built a practice and it is one of the first practices around. I left the practice and reinvented myself.*

- *Way back – passing exams and being a full fledged pediatrician. Passed boards. Getting accepted to medical school.*

- *The day I got my MD.*

- *I don't think about it like that.*

- *Running my own business and making ends meet.*

- *I don't have any one specific moment.*

- *Rather than an individual moment I enjoy patients who have been through the mill of seeing specialist after specialist and failing to get better and then seeing tremendous changes in my practice. Also within the practice of family medicine the ability to extrapolate the path they may take if they continue on their same course and working together to bend the curve to avoid some of the particularly bad outcomes.*

- *It's long forgotten. I have proud moments all the time. I can't really store them. I have done a lot more good than bad in my life.*

- *The moment I realized that I need to be humble.*

- *A lot of little proud moments along the way.*

- *I haven't had a long enough career to feel that one moment stood out than others. I am proud when people get back to normal lives and feel good and don't feel like a health problem defines them.*

- *Because I was involved in teaching and education I have had an opportunity to mold other physicians' careers. That is really gratifying. Helping colleagues and people in training.*

- *Not only one. When I am able to produce work that could be in a textbook. I want everyone to be able to be seen by any doctor and what I did is appreciated as appropriate and good.*

- *There was a patient who was deemed to be terminally ill. I sensed that there was still potential for improvement and I pushed the envelope for her to turn around and get the necessary supportive care. She made it through and went through her daily life, got her hair done and crocheted.*

- *I see children and adults. I saw a woman who was a school librarian and she was in pain and one of the students noticed and said, "If you go see my doctor she will know what to do to fix you." And she came to see me.*

- *I am proud of the fact that I am regarded by my peers as a good doctor. I am a doctors' doctor and I have doctors from the hospital in my practice. I have received awards. I have appointments at the hospital. These accolades are nice. I am appreciated by peers.*

Misc
- *I don't have one per se.*
- *Every day.*

Q: WHAT DID YOU DO AS A DOCTOR THAT REALLY MADE A DIFFERENCE?

* More on the caring, as well as clinical skills of doctoring. It's all intertwined and hard, if not impossible, to separate.

• *Help people over the years. Extend life or help them to deal with some kind of condition that will cut their life short.*

• *Community service, medical practice*

• *I have taken good care of people. Good diagnoses and made a difference in outcomes. I made some mistakes but mostly did well.*

• *I try to make small differences every day in each and every patient I see. Just talking to them about their health or something that is going on in their personal life. Just talking even if not related to health makes a difference.*

• *Being in primary care I don't often have the opportunity to be that guy that the person says, he cut my tumor out of me or did heart surgery that saved my life. But they say if it wasn't for me they wouldn't have found my heart problems. A lot of the things that really make a difference go unnoticed. Quit smoking or change diet. In the long run I had the most effect on people but their ego completely unrecognized it.*

• *I do that all the time. That's what I do. I see critically ill people in the hospital and figure it out when no one else can do it. The people can walk out of the hospital and live without the hospital. I can cure it and they never worry about it again. I love my subspecialty even after all the BS.*

• *So many times when I feel that I have eased my patients' pains in some way. Dealing with crises. I am not an ER doc calling out lab orders. But I will be there and comfort the patients.*

- *Just again, listen to every patient. touched them and really more than making diagnosis, was reassuring them that what they had was not serious and was self limiting. Taking them off half of the medicine that the specialist put them on. It was making them sick.*

- *I took the message and made it more palliative. I have helped parents with the garbage that is out there. I am good at diagnosis with curious cases and communicating information that helps them because I am cutting through the garbage on the internet.*

- *The patients know that if they need me I am there. One patient I have known for 20 years. He had a disorder that was very difficult to diagnose. I was only a resident at that time. So when I had my own practice somehow he knew and he found me. I was seeing him every day in the ICU for three months. It wasn't a five minute visit. He told me years later that seeing me come in and sit and talk to him helped him get better. But, it was very draining on me.*

- *Ask my patients. Saving lives of premature babies. Especially preemies, but sick patients in general who could have died.*

- *I have seen a lot of patients for free.*

- *I don't know that I would know that answer. I have taken women afraid of the doctor and brought them to not be afraid. Women that I have seen for the first time will never be afraid again. One woman: I am really worried about my drinking. She cried. She brought it up with her primary care doctor and he put her on Lexapro.*

- *I don't think about it. Twenty patients out of 25 will say thank you on the way out and probably mean it. For them I am making a difference. It is not obviously every day.*

- *Giving a shoulder to cry on when no one else listened.*

- *Hopefully improving people's lives.*

- *I help people deal with difficult diagnosis or treatment by listening to them thinking about their problems and seeking help when it is the right thing to do.*

- *Teach other doctors, residents, students, and my patients.*

- *One of the things that we spend a lot of time trying to teach the residents and students is to develop their communication skills. Talking and listening. It is very important for the physician to pick up on the anxieties that are paramount to the patient and the family and do their best to address them. Most of the trainees do appreciate and get that. Some are better than others. It has to be a focus on that and lifelong learning. There is too much information. You cannot know all information all the time. Need a base, but also need a lifelong learning plan, so that they can evaluate new information and data and apply it to successfully taking care of patients.*

- *A lot of what I do. I am all over the place.*

- *A whole range of answers to that. Knowing that someone comes with an acute emergency, then doing a simple procedure and they feel great. They think you are terrific. I do more advanced procedures with people who are critically ill or have infections. Sometimes it's dramatic. I have the opportunity to actually do things. When a patient comes to you and you are the fourth and fifth one they have been to and already have a lot of tests and the doctors are sick of them. I sit down and talk to them and I don't give up and they keep coming back and they know you are trying and finally you find something and it makes a difference. You listened. Many of them of have psychological stuff. Compliments make you feel good.*

- *Safely seeing people through a health problem. No one thing.*

- *Hard to say. I think that I make a difference by changing people's expectations of a visit. I also like to think that I have a big impact on patients and end of life care. I try to encourage them to think about it now, not when it is upon them. Death is part of life, no sense beating around the bush.*

- *Easing pain and suffering in other people. Enabling people to die with dignity.*

- *Help people over the years. Extend life or help them to deal with some kind of condition that will cut their life short.*

- *Making people better. Doing what I am trained to do. One patient walked up to me years later and said she thinks of me every day. I am very focused. Another one said that her daughter is doing well. It makes me proud to make a difference. Until you get that feedback, you just don't know.*

- *There isn't one single thing. It's just every little daily detail. Especially in my field. Correcting serious problems and they feel better. When someone is almost at the verge of death and we turn it around.*

- *I would like to hope that I make a difference in a lot of my patients' outcomes when they cooperate. All good doctors make a difference.*

* The doctor patient relationship is so important to the doctor interviewees.

- *Basically I like human relationships with some of my patients.*

- *I stayed with a family when they had to unhook their family member from life support. And when they lost her, I stayed with them and that really made a difference.*

- *What I do makes a difference. I take care of people who people don't care to take care of any more. I also take care of a lot of easy people too.*

- *It's different now days than it was 25 or 30 years ago. I would have said then that I picked up a disease or made a great diagnosis. This is the rubric example, if one is not a surgeon. Picking up something subtle that no one else saw. That doesn't do it for me anymore. It's what we have been trained to do. To me, it's when I help people with lifestyle issues and really helping them with their lives. Not smoking, exercise. When they feel better about themselves and they can attribute it back to our relationship.*

- *In those moments when people are really sick or at the end of life to be there for families. People verbalize that I make a big difference. A million small things that I never realize. That last moment is always remembered. So that being present at that time. Those words that you choose at that moment will resonate with that family for a long time.*

Q: WHAT WAS YOUR LOWEST POINT IN YOUR CAREER AS A DOCTOR?

* Sometimes it was business issues.

- *Leaving a group. I was disappointed and went into solo practice. It turned out to be good.*

- *Business aspect of medicine. I don't like it, I don't want to do it, I don't like it I don't want to do it. You have to change.*

- *I lost partners. It's very upsetting. People leave. There are all kinds of issues.*

- *The point where we affiliated with a practice management organization and I thought that we were going to lose our practice.*

- *Dealing with bureaucrats who don't know it and don't care and dealing with people whose motivation is profit and don't admit it.*

- *Obamacare*

* Lawsuits are an incredible low point for my interviewees. As one said, "Being made to feel like I did something wrong when I really didn't."

- *I had received a lawsuit. It turned to be nothing and the case got dropped. But I was young and I didn't know anything about it; my heart dropped and I was in a state of anxiety and depression for months; a person who walked in without an appointment and was complaining about mild chest discomfort radiating to the left arm. The EKG was different than his last one and I faxed the results to his cardiologist. Waiting for the cardiologist to call. It took about an hour. I didn't have the old EKG. I faxed it to the cardiologists to compare it. It came back and it had changed and we sent him to the ER and he had a stroke, not a heart attack, and he sued me for delay of care. The chart had been sent out to many lawyers and nobody took it and his own son was representing him. I was young and I didn't know anything about it. I had insomnia. I didn't go to work. They were even unable to get an affidavit of merit to pay an expert. Completely frivolous. The son took the case to just keep his parents happy. Ruined my life for six months.*

- *I had a couple of malpractice cases over the years. It always just knocks your stomach out. Every day I make decisions that could come back and be judged in another light. One little thing happens and escalates with other things. Every day we have to make decisions and choices and sometimes it doesn't come out right and that hurts. But shit happens. It hurts, I am not in the business to not have things work out. It sucks. That is the closest that I felt to being depressed. Lost joy in life. I am usually very joyous. Appreciative. Looking back I would make the same choice even though what happened doesn't usually happen. It takes your joy out.*

- *A malpractice case. Five years after I saw a patient, I got subpoenaed that I missed the diagnosis. Her exam was so benign. I sent her for an x-ray. There was nothing on exam. So years later, the x-ray came back as a fracture. The first case was thrown out. Second malpractice suit. The woman said that I made her scared of cancer for the rest of her life. She had no insurance, etc. I said that she needed a biopsy. It was all documented. It was a shock that someone would sue me. It went to trial. My insurance company asked me to settle. I thought that it was my fault. We ended up in court. It took me out of my schedule for as much time I was in court. They sued the other doctor too.*

- *I was sued. They didn't collect. I had to go to court. They claimed I missed a diagnosis. This one I missed. But then he was okay anyway. It was 20 years ago.*

- *We get sued, even though we won. It still sucked. We had an elderly lady in a nursing home and the family was pissed off. They went to a lawyer. We spent two weeks in court. We won but it was awful.*

- *I'm in the middle of a lawsuit right now. I just got the plaintiff's expert report. It is completely idiotic. No end in sight and it has gone on for three years. It makes me feel lousy. I saw the patient once in 2008 and he was fine. And the patient died in 2012 and out of my care. Makes you second guess yourself. I had a patient I actually helped who did badly. I called the wife yesterday; he died at home. I feel bad because I was especially close with the patient and family. The malpractice suits are the lowest points. I had another one 10 years ago. These are bad things. The patient had a rare but known complication. Ninety-nine percent of the time you don't get sued. When it is genuine, I understand. Sometimes I wonder, why do I really still want to do it? Then you need another experience to salvage it. Most days I still want to still do it. For this particular case, I don't feel a lot of responsibility. It makes people like me a little bitter and it definitely creates defensive medicine.*

- *A couple of mistakes. One in residency. One time I almost got sued. An error of not being assertive enough. I have a problem with that. I have to remind myself to listen to the voice, if someone else says no and I know it's right. I feel partially responsible. I learned from it.*

- *I settled one suit. I have a friend who is a malpractice lawyer who said that if I went to trial I would have a 90 percent chance of winning, but we settled. It's truly miserable, even the preparation. I couldn't imagine actually being in a courtroom for however many days.*

- *Being sued. It was a severely premature pregnancy with complications. I first met the woman when she was already in labor. After a few hours I was unable to stop the labor. She delivered and the baby died. I was sued for wrongful death.*

- *Being deposed. Being made to feel like I did something wrong when I really didn't. The ability to fabricate a case out of something nonexistent. Saying that you have deviated from a standard, but you didn't. I have another one now. The patient said I did something and we have electronic confirmation that the patient wasn't even here that day.*

- *The second time I got sued. It was a case I had. I was moonlighting in an urgent care center. A guy came in with really vague symptoms. He had seen a doctor the day before. He had a pain in his chest, not classic for a heart attack. Twenty minutes after he left my clinic he keeled over from a heart attack. I called the covering MD. I knew I would be sued. The jury determined in my favor after an hour. That was years later. In the meantime there was a tremendous amount of angst and soul searching.*

- *When I went to a legal situation where a doctor with whom I had a financial disagreement made up falsehoods about how I practice.*

- *I was falsely accused in a job and I was let go for medical malpractice.*

- *My one and only malpractice suit. It was ridiculous. I was found not guilty but it made me really question whether I should continue to practice medicine.*

- *A very traumatic experience and a confrontation with the hospital that involved litigation and eventually it got resolved, although not entirely and fairly, and I had to accept it. They had concocted something that was about to ruin my reputation and I had to fight back. It made me think, do I really even want to be a doctor?*

- *I had one lawsuit after 30 years of practice. It was horrible. I had to settle. I took care of four generations of his family. He was diabetic, never compliant and never did what he was supposed to do. He had rectal bleeding. We made an appointment right here in my office for a colonoscopy and he didn't go. I had to settle. He got $600,000. That dragged on for three years. It was horrible.*

* Our doctors are people too. They have personal lives, complete with stress, just like the rest of us. They have feelings about their lives, just like the rest of us

Q: HOW DID YOU FEEL ABOUT IT?

- *When my nanny was having a stroke and I was very early in my career. I handled it pretty good. Found a good nanny who has been with me for six years.*

- *The sexism in my training and at the hospital. I did not let it deter me. It was a real handicap. There is no equality. Do not be independent and successful.*

- *Third year of residency with 112 hours a week working. I dated a professor. It was wonderful until it wasn't. I was set up with the man I married. He never forgave me for getting on with my life. The other residents asked why he was so brutal to me. He was awkward toward me or undercut me. I had family members hospitalized and one of them died on my wedding day. I had exams. They told me not to study, but everyone else did. The others did better. Sixty-six percent% versus 99 percent. I was labeled as the stupid one. They told me they wouldn't support me. A dark six months for me. Next year I studied my ass off and they finally decided that I wasn't an idiot.*

- *My chief in surgery called me in and said that I don't have the personality of the surgeon. He said, don't get involved in tangential issues, like social, the endocrine, and other issues. After three years I was dropped from general surgery department. I got hired as a surgeon and I worked for 15 years there and got better experience. I was a house surgeon.*

* Patient care is often stressful and packed with feelings.

- *Losing an 8 year old boy who was a little sick, but had toxic shock syndrome and died later that night. I had a nagging moment of should I have seen it.*

- *Watching a 23 year old boy with incurable disease die.*

- *When I had accidents that could have been avoided and that impacted the health of the patients. I was sued. A few times. I was very impacted emotionally. But I didn't consider it the lowest point. It was a frivolous situation. At times I have made real errors but I found plenty of compassion from my patients.*

- *Any time you lose somebody. It's inevitable, but when someone dies and you know the family that is the pretty much where it is.*

- *I might lose it on you. Maybe 14 years ago. My cousin. I loved her. I was her doctor. She had complications after a procedure. She went into a coma and she died a week later. It was awful. No contact with that part of the family again. It was my husband's friend; my kids' friends. I went to therapy and I was in therapy for a couple of years. I couldn't do that procedure for awhile, then I got a wonderful letter from another doctor and I was able to do it again. The husband didn't sue me. We had a meeting and talked. When I look back medically, I did everything I could do but it wasn't enough. Now I am affiliated with a medical center that offers immediate emergency help to try and prevent these sorts of events.*

- *I have many low points. I take it seriously if I missed something when a patient passed away and I could have stopped it.*

- *When I haven't been present or haven't listened and I missed something that was important because I was in a hurry to get to the next patient or the next part of my day.*

Misc

- *Not too many.*
- *Always ups and downs. No particular event.*

Q: What was your most difficult experience or hardest day as a doctor?

* Of course there are business and insurance issues.

- *I expected to be around tough and hard cases. I expected it to be hard. I did not expect to have to think if the insurance company will not pay for it.*
- *A lot. Examples: deaths. Some of the procedures can have complications even if you do nothing wrong but the patient is worse off than before. A couple of cases where it went to lawsuits and you have to sit in a courtroom and list to what an SOB you are and you have to defend yourself. There were no deviations from protocol, but it was injurious. This was a low point.*

* The clinical work load can be demanding.

- *The hardest day is when I am up all night, next day have big surgeries and then the afternoon or evening I have to see 30-40 patients.*
- *It is hard when I am really tired and have to think. I found out I was hypothyroid and understood why this was happening.*
- *First year of internship. It was all so new to me.*

* Patient deaths, again, so hard to bear.

- *The first time I had information for a family of a loved one's cancer and death.*

- *Losing a patient who I was very attached to for many years.*

- *During my residency there were three or four deaths in a 24-hour period. That was my hardest day.*

- *In residency as a second year resident we were in charge of running codes, and two codes in particular stick out as particularly challenging for me. A woman coded after a complicated C section of her 3rd baby. We coded her 7-8 times and she seemed to get better, went to the ICU had a massive cerebral hemorrhage and died. As the 3rd year resident a 22 year old school teacher with a UTI with 24 hours full blown sepsis, she walked in and then in 3 hours coded. I was supervising the residents and she died anyway. I gave my residents the good job speech and went home and cried.*

- *The most horrible death I had ever witnessed with patient. I felt like I had messed up. Most problems were alcohol or drugs. Some things we had never seen before. One patient died and it was horrible.*

- *Watching young people die.*

- *In my training I had a 20-year-old boy come in with a virus that attacked his system very quickly and within 24 hours he was dead. I was with the family. The absolute most difficult was 9/11 and we prepared an ICU and no one showed up. I would have been better as a welder or a fireman. It was the only time I ever felt useless as a doctor.*

- *When I still cannot come to terms with the care of terminally ill patients. Not one, in general. As a doctor you are called to correct things and sometimes things are not correctable.*

- *I had a patient in the hospital with an irreversible neuromuscular disease. She was on a breathing tube and said, "I do not want to live anymore." I discussed with her parents and her minister, and we all agreed it was time to unplug her. It was in 1990. I went to the funeral and spoke. She was 18.*

- *Final moments of saying good bye to a patient that I have taken care of, diagnosed, and been with all along. For example, I had one patient with pancreatic cancer who died in 7 months.*

* Very sick patients may have been saved, but working with them was still packed with feelings.

- *I will always remember this. Massive bleeding during a surgery. Other doctors and I saved the patient's life.*

- *As an intern I had four admissions. All four were septic. If your Blood Pressure was low, you were put on meds. In the real world you only do it in the ICU. We used to do it on the floor. Now there are monitors that control the rate of the flow so you know what you are doing. In the old days, you could adjust the flow rate and a watch and a drip and adjust. It was hard.*

- *Today. I have a very sick patient and I had to go in the middle of the night.*

- *Not one hardest day. When someone dies. As a physician I have become very good at compartmentalizing things. In a patient room, office, or hospital and that person and family is the most important and then you have to more on and the next person is the most important. If you dwell on someone having a hard time or passing way it is the hardest.*

- *When I was still seeing kids, I had a 9-year-old diagnosed with a brain tumor.*

* Giving patients bad news is also packed with feelings.

- *Telling a family bad news. This happened 15 years ago. I had done a surgery on the patient. Of all procedures it was one of the most dangerous. It seemed uneventful and he seemed okay, but he died during the night. I had to explain it and console them. They did not sue me. The problem with malpractice is if you have a good victim and they look pitiable and there is a lot of money involved it becomes a business decision. Settled cases go on your database and court as if you lost. Somehow you think that it reflects on you.*

- *Giving people terminal illness diagnoses.*

- *Having to tell someone who had an unanticipated health issue that it would not improve and that they would have to live with it.*

- *Long forgotten. Too many, such as when you have to give a patient bad news.*

- *The most difficult experience is imparting life changing news. I like interacting with people. It's not hard to stay up all night.*

- *When the patient is angry or leaves the practice and you know they left because they are angry or when you have to break bad news to a patient. I had one today. That is tough. I had one today and one eight months ago. I got the results on a Friday night and I knew that he wanted to know. I called him up and I said I know what I thought was going on and I do not want you to go on the internet. Those are tough. When you lose a friend or when a patient who has been close to you dies it's tough. Usually that is more a chronic thing that you are going through with them. Usually when there is a dying patient at least as a family doctor there are things you can do to help. So you don't feel helpless.*

Misc
- *No one biggest one.*

Q: What was your biggest disappointment as a doctor?

* Business and insurance issues are ever present and so disappointing. This is not medicine or patient care, which is what they trained to do. It is not what they expected or wanted.

- *To struggle to make ends meet in this day and age.*

- *The amount of time that I have to spend behind the scenes with administration stuff making things happen. It takes away from the time I can spend with my patients. Insurance, logistics etc. I can't just walk away.*

- *The administration and how they run everything.*

- *Changes in the system and the need for forming a group*

- *Obamacare.*

- *The intrusions that our health care system has had on time and patient relationships. I was sued once when I was in first in practice. It was dismissed. Summary dismissal. 1978. Stressful but over quickly. Biggest stress is pushing away all of the intrusions so that I can spend time with the patient I do a lot of the paperwork and BS afterwards they leave. I do not sit with a computer. They have my full attention.*

- *Being taken over by a bigger practice. Can't be a small business.*

- *I guess I thought I would have been retired by this time and that my income would not have dropped so radically over the years.*

- *In practice it is more about being a business person than a doctor.*

- *Watching the development of the system that we have today. The abusive patients. The lack of listening. Doctors don't listen to the patients who then listen to their computers. The dichotomy of billing. Overbilling the patients because it is a third party system. The insurance system underpays, so nowhere is there reality in the entire system. Also an overwhelming amount of overbilling and over collection passed on to physicians. Hospitals, medical suppliers, pharmaceutical houses, and insurance companies get payments, as opposed to physicians getting payments. Clean up the facility charges. If we could solve the Medicaid problem we could solve the whole problem. EMTALA is law 30 years old. Every hospital must treat every patient who walks into the door. We should have a triage system like the Cleveland Clinic. Send people to the Marriot instead of $3,000 a day for being in the hospital. I would put together a panel of doctors and have utilization review versus quality control. There are so many things that we could do to be cost effective. Add all of that and give us tort reform.*

- *The abrupt closing of one of our offices for financial reasons that could have been avoided. It's happening in about 10 days. It's a shame.*

- *Malpractice is a big disappointment. When you get to a certain age you realize that you can't do everything or be an expert in everything. Have to accept what you time constraints and job setting is and etc. We are now affiliated with a hospital. We can't just do our jobs.*

- *What became enjoyable to me was to talk with people. I partnered with a clinical psychologist. How could I bill*

*for it? I couldn't do it. I was "the slow one." Sometimes I
still have nightmares about not having enough time. I was
always told that I was never working up to my potential. I
feel like that.*

- *A lot of doctors are not very nice. Money becomes too much
the issue. I am disappointed that more people are not in
favor of single payer. It bothers me that people blame the
government for so many of the problems of the things we
have to do when it is insurance companies.*

- *Most people go into medicine to help people. Meet the
bureaucrats and people looking to make money and that is
the biggest one. It bugs me.*

- *To see how the sanctity of the doctor-patient relationship
is being destroyed. I think the doctor-patient relationship
has been violated by the interference of third parties of all
natures. Politicians are looking for power, and insurance
companies endorsed by politicians are looking for money and
power, and lawyers are looking for profit.*

- *The biggest continuing problem is the administrative burden
placed on us and the continuous demand to see more and
more patients. I am on a commission and there is one
resolution about physician burnout. Deal with the root
cause, which is that we have to see too many patients and
too much paperwork.*

- *Associates come and go. It's disappointing and adds stress
to call schedules.*

- *Commercialization and corporatization of medicine.*

- *The amount of time we spend on paperwork and systems
issues as opposed to patient care. Authorization for meds
and not even a third line experimental medication. Something
that is first line that they can benefit from. Maybe we can*

get it but it is hours of phone calls, paperwork and triage. Beats the patient and healthcare team down. Most doctors and residents want to do what is best for the patients and work very hard at trying to do that. Same way the patients want to do what is best for them. Patient perspective; there is so much information out there bombarding patients. Internet lookup and being bombarded with stories. Good but also causes information overload and I have seen it generate a lot of anxiety. Worry about patients and healthcare workers gets distracting and there is tangential from information on the internet. Some things are straightforward, but do not want to get distracted. A strep throat needs an antibiotic to knock it out. It does not need a lot of research.

* Patient relationships and care can be disappointing.

• *When I couldn't make a difference. When I realized that I couldn't fix everything.*

• *Personally, not having the freedom to care for patients as thoroughly as I would like to do. Sometimes that means time. Sometimes that means money. And seeing my patients seeing other doctors not take care of them like I think they need to be taken care of or pushed through the system. Understanding that as a physician I am sacrificing my family for yours. My dad is gone now for seven years I couldn't save him, but I have to save your family every day.*

• *Once a year when I have to tell parents that their child is dying and there is nothing I can do to stop it. I hate giving people news like this, but I am not going to lie. I went to his wake and funeral. I stayed in close touch with the family.*

• *When there is still a bad outcome even when you try to do what you can with everything you can with, all of your knowledge, but sometimes things just don't go their way.*

Lowest point. You cannot leave this job. Family is secondary. No real peace, everything is always on. Can't ignore certain things. Can't plan too far in advance out of the blue. I have not been sued.

- *When my mother died. Everyone in my family was looking to me to make a miracle happen. I thought that I was a failure. I think that she knew that I was right and she died in my arms.*

* Negative patient behavior, in spite of best efforts on the part of the doctor, can be disappointing

- *Feeling disappointment. Dealing with a Borderline Personality Disorder patient. She has two elderly parents. She is on disability and blah blah blah. But she is taking care of her parents. She wasn't my active patient at the time although I had seen her over the years. I empathize with her. One day, busy day, I always call her back, I take extra time, I squeeze them in. One day she gives me this beautiful gift she made me. Then it's a Monday, she calls, I am triple booked, it's crazy. She called about her father, another doctor in our practice took the call. She ended up cursing me out at the end of our conversation. "I am so disappointed in you." A few months later I said let's move on.*

- *In my previous practice. I was so naïve. I was just out of medical school. I was taken advantage of because I wanted to be so open and so accessible.*

- *An example is someone who you really go out of your way to help and they end up turning against you and badmouth you to other people. I personally may have a tendency of overestimating some people in terms of thinking that they will appreciate what I am doing and maybe overextending, and then their interpretation of it becomes negative. It's a disappointment that they don't appreciate it. Maybe it was a misjudgment on my part. I tend to be naïve and think the best of people.*

* Business or practice issues, as always, can be disappointing.

• *I am doubly board certified and they wouldn't give me my permanent hospital privileges. I had to hire a lawyer and then it went away. It was awful.*

• *I wish I could be faster. Think faster. Make the diagnoses faster. Type faster. I don't want my patients to wait, but I always run late. They know that but they still bitch.*

• *I don't recall being disappointed. Some trivial things, like people not showing up for office hours. Missing a diagnosis. Nothing financial. None of my kids became doctors.*

• *None of my kids want to be dealing with illness.I cry or hug my partner and hug my husband who is a doctor. If I go back to work, I feel better when I am upset. I go to the next case and try to make a difference.*

• *I am happy overall being a doctor. Over diagnosis is a problem. As physicians we are medically and legally obligated to order all sort of things that will never kill a patient but will cause tremendous stress. For me too, what if I missed something?*

• *Mostly it's been positive.*

Misc
• *Not too many.*
• *Can't think of one.*

Q: WHAT WAS YOUR BIGGEST STRESS AS A DOCTOR? HOW DID YOU HANDLE IT?

* Lawsuits are very stressful. As one doctor said, "I felt violated."

• *To be held responsible for what I can't control. If they don't do as I told them it's my fault. The malpractice system is also very frustrating.*

• *The deposition. I felt violated. I just got through it.*

• *Fear of being sued. You do everything you can but there are always multiple ways to look at it. There are not many joys left in medicine. You can always have a job. Besides money you want people to get better and appreciate it. Don't get paid a lot of money per hour. Patients are more selfish and greedy. Start to get an edge and are always on guard. Even with honest patients, I always wonder what their motive is and then you get burned. When I first came out it is totally different. Handling the office and the practice. Financially keeping all of the employees happy and motivating them to do their best every day. A big part of it. Sometimes the patients are easier. Insurance company business is a bigger part of the day.*

• *The malpractice suits. I used to work every other Saturday, 9am-6pm days. They are stressful, but it didn't bother me and at the end of the day it was an accomplishment. The work stuff never bothered me.*

• *Right now I feel like a lot of it is all the non patient related stuff that is being forced upon us. Electronic Medical Records all of the extra documentation that is being required for Medicare, Meaningful Use, Accountable Care Organizations And there is a certain fear that goes on that every patient who walks in the door is a potential lawsuit. That is a real risk. It's tough. I handle it as best I can by trying to get everything done and I try to have a good rapport with my patients and practice good medicine and trying to be obsessive compulsive about it.*

- *In addition to insurance stress and being taken over by a big practice, being on call. I don't get annoyed though if it's a real need.*

- *Being sued twice. I have won both. The stress was horrible, staying up at night wondering what I did wrong. The first one the jury dropped immediately. The second one was being sued by an evangelical minister. I took care of him for free for 15 years. He sued me and my wife. He didn't get a colonoscopy when we told him to get one, so he got colon cancer. They couldn't get any expert witnesses against me. I took care of him for free and his wife.*

- *Making ends meet. Dealing with increasing costs of running a business versus diminishing returns.*

- *The incident that I mentioned earlier with medical malpractice defenses. I tend to handle stress. I don't pay as much attention to personal stress management. I orient towards the source and resolve it. With the hospital it was to fight it.*

Q: How did you feel about it?

- *It's hopeless. No hope in that we are looked on by people, government and agencies as the bad person.*

- *It can be overwhelming. It can be very crippling at times. To make sure that you are spending time with other things all the while when there is a lot of this other stuff like insurance companies refusing to approve a drug that the patient has been on for years and is doing well with.*

- *For some doctors, certainly to me, I have some object around being a good doctor. I tend to have my self esteem as a high quality doctor and doing the right thing. A certain amount of pride around it. When it gets assaulted my reaction can be strong. Depressed, angry, or fighting back. If your self esteem is predominately based around an internal point immune to criticism. If it is external then you become vulnerable. For me some of mine is around pride of the high quality of doctor that I am. When that gets assaulted it becomes very distressing. Get real and say I am who I think I am. Don't be so vulnerable to the plaintiff's attorney, the hospital committee, the irate family member or patient. Easier said than done.*

* Business and practice issues are stressful. Sometimes there is a solution, or at least a partial solution.
- *Not had much stress. Handled time expectations with coverage every other night and weekend. I got on a bicycle and rode, which I still do.*
- *Surgeons are like fighter pilots and Marine leaders. We rise to stress.*

* Sometimes there is no readily available reasonable solution. As one interviewee said, "Throw me in jail, if you must, for taking care of a child whose parent cannot afford to pay. What jail do they have for doctors who care too much?" Others also struggled with no readily available solution.
- *Working long intense hours at times.*
- *I unfortunately am the economic engine for this practice and my family so I have to wake up and hit the ground running. The nature of my practice is such is that I could be busier*

but the quality of my work would be different. Not disease based or market driven. Have to contend with different rules than the average doctor. I could do more office work and less surgery. Market forces are brutal.

- *There are days when there is too much going on. Everyone is making demands and too much. Sometimes I snap at the staff or short with the patients so I try and take a deep breath. I always feel remorse. Hard to apologize but I make myself do it.*

- *Stress is increased in our society as a whole and it is no different in healthcare, for the patients and the providers. It manifests in the residency training programs. One of the biggest stressors is the competing demands in limited time, which is hard for residents, MD's and nurses. There is an increasing body of medical knowledge and technology that everyone has to be familiar with. There is an increasing number of patients that one is expected to see within an increasingly bureaucratic system.*

- *The students and residents are very concerned about the debt that they have accumulated over their years of training. Some have over $100-$200k. Those going into primary care have lower salaries than those going into specialties. Sometimes that drives some young doctors away from primary care fields to more specialized areas.*

- *Time. I handled it by getting to work earlier and staying later.*

- *It's frustrating. I did try to stick to the schedule. I hated it when I kept people waiting.*

- *Dealing with partners who are greed driven. I ignore them, exercise, and meditate. They are not worth my anger and destroying my health.*

- *The time crunch. Just to be able to do everything that I want to do and need to do. I want to do everything. I like what I do. I couldn't do anything else. I'd like to do less of it, but my days are getting longer and longer and it is a stress. I don't want to just work.*

- *Not having enough time to do the work, to read, to keep up. All of that.*

- *When I graduated residency, I had a vision of what kind of practice I wanted to have. It didn't involve joining a big practice or a hospital. I wanted to be my own boss and do it the way I wanted to do it. Building a business from scratch and in about eight months, but I did not have enough patients to be sure. If not for my wife I would have joined a big practice. There is a lot of financial stress.*

- *I realize how many people count on me and depend on me. Not just the patients. The office staff and my partners keep me awake worrying. For example, the new lease. The rent quadruples. Every time I make a decision I feel that anxiety. Will this work? How will it affect everyone? So far I have been okay. I ruminate and stress and do calculations again and again. It's getting worse and worse. The insurance companies. Even when they agree to pay we wait two-and-a-half years for reimbursement. It's getting more and more pervasive, the problems in reimbursement. I can't tell someone no. Throw me in jail, if you must, for taking care of a child whose parent cannot afford to pay. What jail do they have for doctors who care too much?*

- *Dealing with all the paperwork, the legislative stuff, the re-certifications, and having to constantly explain my billing to the insurance companies and Medicare.*

* Patient care is often difficult and stressful.

• *Hard to diagnose patients. I keep trying.*

• *After years of practicing, having to do a devastating emergency surgery because of bleeding problems of the patient. I had long and serious conversations with the patient and her husband. I felt sad.*

• *Being a doctor you have to realize no matter how good you are at diagnostic meds, or prevention, there is no guarantee that the patient will not die. It's tough. It's hard sometimes. I take death as a personal affront. I work hard to keep you going, it's not fair. I talk to God and the angel of death all the time. Cut the patient a break give them a little more time and make them better.*

• *Staying on 100 percent. Keeping my mind and merging the things that I told you about earlier. Ultimately I need to make the right decision for the patient: No allergy, no drug-to-drug interaction. That it's the right thing to pick and still have a smile on my face, be pleasant, be empathetic. Trying to figure out the unspoken things that they are not telling me. All the while staying on time. Dealing with patients complaints. 90-95 percent are amazing. A few of them are complaining. Even if it's only been five minutes although they came an hour early and say they have been there for an hour.*

• *It was always patient load and making sure I didn't make mistakes with critically ill patients with so much responsibility. I handled it one patient at a time. Having multiple critically ill patients in the hospital and having to deal with several sicknesses at one time with too many patients.*

• *Biggest stress was long hours and patients' waiting time, when that was their biggest complaint. It was a killer. No matter what I did I could never get ahead. Doctors now spend more and more time treating and seeing well patients and getting treated better for treating well patients than sick patients. We would have very sick patient come in when it was time to go home. Today you go to the ER.*

- *Always being worried that you are going to do something wrong or harmful.*

Misc
- *None that I can recall.*

* Personal issues are stressful, as they are for all of us.

- *Going through three years of fellowship and three nannies. Starting my first job and going through six nannies in six months.*

- *When I had postpartum depression. I got the help and got back on track. That was the worst year.*

- *Finding a balance between work and the kids. Having time for the kids. Can't distinguish work and doctor. It's kind of like who you are. As a medical student I used to look at the attending and see your identity is your profession. This weekend I am on call and my son's car broke down.*

- *It is almost a daily thing. You deal with decisions of life and death. My faith has a lot to do with it. The other day as I was waiting for the elevator after Psalm 21 came to mind and that encouraged me. I lift up my eyes. My wife and children have been extremely encouraging. I cannot do it without their daily encouragement.*

- *That's how I handle it. My faith. A doctor's job is very unique. In the same hour you could see a convict who needs help in finding a place in society and refill meds and needs help reentering society, and the next patient could be superior court judge. Medicine levels the playing field.*

*Treat everyone as VIP and you cannot go wrong. The
spectrum of things that you treat may seem trivial. For
example, an 84-year-old lady who is tired and having hair
loss but that is important. In the next moment you are
dealing with someone who cannot decide if he wants further
hospice care or to go on chemo, writing an excuse for work
or jury duty to signing a death certificate.*

Q: WHAT DOES THE JOB ENTAIL?

* The responses are the same: it is a combination of
clinical skills and caring.

• *Time and effort.*

• *Being smart, compulsive and compassionate.*

• *Compassion and understanding, especially with anxious
new mothers, especially new infant care.*

• *I see patients when they are well, have well patients,
sometimes I do surgeries, sometimes I do other procedures.*

• *It's a fascinating job. It is never dull. Every single patient
is different, even if they have the same diagnosis. You never
know what you will see or do before you go into the room
and interact. In an hour you can deal with everything from
every corner of the textbook. It is exciting and stressful, it is
difficult to remember all of the facts, to have to look up drugs,
etc. Needing to be right all the time, which is impossible.
You can't do it you can just try and hard and then correct
things. You have to juggle all the facts. You have to apply
them to his person who may or may not be telling you the
whole story correctly and may have their own issues. Medicine
is less of a science than people think, although it is based
in science. We don't understand everything. People have a
symptom and we cannot give them a diagnosis maybe ever.*

Not every symptom has a reason. It is hard. And there is an ever increasing data base of information. So many guidelines are often conflicting and what the patient wants and what the system thinks they want are often in conflict. We are the patients' advocate but you are also the systems gatekeepers and those two are sometimes in conflict. For example, if I have an atypical symptom, do I do a potentially unnecessary test, or if I say no, will I be sued? Have to go through preauthorization and plead the cases. It happens more and more with meds.

- *A lot of work. A lot of work. Now it's a crazy amount of work.*

- *Everything. Which is growing exponentially and with all of the quality stuff, which some of it is good but there are so many things that we need to do. Some causes us to practice better, but a lot of it is just spinning our wheels so that we can document. Running a business. Run a small business in the health care industry. Keeping people healthy.*

- *Perseverance.*

- *A lot of stress, a lot of learning to have to catch up* with *work and to be re-certified.*

Q: WHY IS IT SO HARD TO BE A DOCTOR? WHAT DOES THE PUBLIC NEED TO UNDERSTAND?

* Surprisingly, "It's not hard to be a doctor." The other aspects, besides the clinical work, are what is hard. Why? Because "This society accepts no mistakes."

- *I'll tell you a story. My first exam in medical school, I got an 80, which was above average. My father said: "Would you want to go to a doctor who is right 80% of the time?" It is the only job where you cannot make a mistake. A lawyer, appeals court, there is none here. It is hard to live up to that standard of being right all the time. People don't realize how much pressure to be right all the time. Nobody's body reads the textbook before they get sick. Gotta be right all the time. Not every case is black and white.*

- *Just like I have misconceptions of patients, people have misconceptions of physicians and there are bad physicians. Most try to do the right thing for patients. There are always those who are more business minded and out for the money. There are physicians who go to sleep thinking about them. Most physicians do care what happens to their patients. They call them at 8pm even thought they should be at their son's baseball game. I am very thorough and don't get paid for it. There are certain things that I do not have to do. And I do it and I don't get paid for it. I have a million phone calls and it is hard to answer all of them. We do the best we can and try and reach out and take care of as much as we can. So hard to be a doctor. This can vary from my standpoint. I am a clinical consultant and I work on what others send me. It's a business but I have to do a good job so people notice and send patients. There's a lot of politics involved and sometimes even if you are very good, you may not get them. There are cliques and hard to find them. I had to take a loan in the beginning. I was running to ten hospitals and two of them closed.*

- *Challenges, responsibilities*

- *I don't think that it is so hard to be a doctor; once you get through medical school and training, you have the skills you need. Need to hone in personality and make it an asset in terms of taking care of people. It is not pure science. It is a lot of intuition and experience. Experience counts a lot because you have seen a lot. Some of your best doctors retire early because they do not want to put up with the BS. It is so intrusive.*

- *It is not hard to be a doctor. It is how you manage your time and communication with your patients. Patients forget that we also have our obligations to our families and cannot get back to them right away and are not always available when they need it. But this is why there is 911 and partners helping us out.*

- *I think that it is hard to be a doctor. Again there is a lot to know. You are expected to know a great deal of information. You are expected to be available 24/7 and you are expected to practice flawless medicine and still get all of the documentation and paperwork done that needs to be done. We are not all millionaires. And in general doctors do what they can do to help patients. A lot of time they are not thought of that way.*

- *New Jersey in 2015. The public and the government expect you to do the impossible. Take care of patients flawlessly with no money. The expectations of America cannot be accomplished. You are going to have morbidity and mortality. Dinging us by taking money away hurts the patient. It makes doctors resentful: I hate the patients and I hate the lawyers. And hate your profession and regret what you are doing. None of us thought it would be like this. You go into it altruistically thinking you will help people, have an interesting life and be financially stable. Working long hours but still, it would be okay. You never think that you will be a Rockefeller but that you will be comfortable. Doctors are pulling their children away from it. Everyone is taking things away, everyone wants a piece of you. You are a lottery ticket to the patients. The lawyers make a ton of money. The insurance companies want you to not spend their money or you are out. The hospitals watch your costs of what you spend. It you spend too much you are dinged.*

And all of this information is given out. It doesn't take into account who the patients are, i.e. nursing home patients. None of this is taken into account. The way that you have to practice medicine now is all about money. How can you work under these conditions? Now every single test that I order has to be put through an insurance company. I am talking to someone who gets paid $12 an hour who makes the decision. One patient now for example. I tried to keep him out of the hospital. But I needed more information. The test had to be pre-certified. It took three weeks. He had bad insurance so he switched to Medicare. It's infuriating. You cannot practice medicine like this. And you have to see enough patients to pay the bills.

• *New health care changes and not having all the answers for patients when they ask about insurance.*

• *This society accepts no mistakes. And in any job that people perform – in any job it will never be 100 percent perfect. The public needs to understand that your whole life is dedicated to caring for patients, putting in long hours, calling patients at night. Dealing with families who are dealing with sick patients and dying patients.*

• *Because medicine is an art, not a science. There is science but there is no binary code. Things are not black and white. No diagnosis is absolute. People want an immediate answer. Things have to play out over time. Plus the business part. And the demanding patients. They want everything. Patients who have the least wrong with them are the most difficult. If they have problems I don't mind the time. Some patients have personality disorders and some have been sexually abused.*

• *The public needs to understand that they do not understand the tests and that they can ask questions and can say no. Patients who refuse a procedure or a test often get dismissed from practice. Don't just give people tests, see what is the problem. We treated patients that day and many of them walked out that day. They need a compassionate doctor who will take care of them.*

- *It is hard to be a doctor today, which is different than 30 years ago when I first started. It was a much nicer relationship with the patients, they trusted me to make decisions with them, not for them, and they knew I was giving them my best and had no motivation except with the best for their child and insurance and the relationship changed a more strained and more adversarial relationship. I always feel that they might sue me. I always was afraid that I would make a mistake. The boy who died, the parents were lawyers, they never sued, they left the sister in the practice. Even in the worst circumstance they did not blame and they trusted me. I believed in the relationship and I felt it was the right thing to do to talk to them. As the years have gone on the doctor-patient relationship has changed. It is not that I chose you because I believe in you and trust you. The public needs to understand that they need to trust the doctors again. There is so much bad and wrong information and criminal information that people believe. They would rather believe a website than believe the doctor who went to medical school and has the experience. They would rather take unscientific information and question and combat the medicine. Everyone thinks that we went into medicine for the money. We went to help people and enjoy the relationship and we get paid with trust and the respect. When that goes it is just stress and paperwork. If people don't shift and come back and appreciate the doctors you will lose your doctor and when you need them the most the people on the internet will not come to the hospital and get you a specialist. There is a lack of respect now and go to a quick easy clinic. It's easier but there is a lack of the whole picture. The pediatrician has known the family for years and picks things up from that knowledge.*

- *I don't think that it's hard to be a doctor if you have the qualities in the first place. If you go into it for the wrong reasons, then it's hard. Any job can be difficult. If you love what you are doing, it's not hard. Tiring, but not hard.*

- *You are dealing with life and death. Every person thinks that they are the most important person in the world. I am triaging all the time. This is more important than that. A 35-year-old with chest pain and 80-year-old mother. Or it's the 50th time you did it today you have to make the person and family feel important but you have to do it all day and all night.*

- *I never felt that it was hard to be a doctor. You should ask first if it's hard. Their doctor is not available 24 hours a day but that there is adequate coverage if it can't wait.*

- *Because you are responsible for things that you can't control. In our society and our culture we need to assume responsibility for ourselves and act like adults.*

- *You give up your twenties. Don't have that play time that all your friends have. It is hard education wise. Residency and then fellowship. I didn't pay off my loans until I was in my 40s. I have a solid job. I'm not poor. My children will not starve. I have relationships with my patients. If their insurance changes they are forced to leave me, I get that. But it interferes with the relationships that used to exist with doctors and patients. We should pay MD's because we value them. Paid directly for service and it is a known value. There is a middle person between us who gets in the way of them by having skin in the game. Also, it pisses me off. If I tell you to get a mammogram and you don't and you have cancer then I am at fault. It should not be my responsibility. Patients are adults. Patients don't take responsibility for their health care like they should. Take more responsibility for your health and do what we tell you to do. We are making these suggestions not for our own good. Lifestyle changes, we have to ask the patients to make reasonable ones. Can't give people too big chunks of what to do.*

- *Other doctors around me are trying to move so fast that they no longer communicate. Among doctors there is a lack of communication. It is difficult and you need to make to make the time to really explain things to people. It is hard to give people plans they can understand*

- *You need to be compulsive, determined, patient, have stamina, be able to step outside of your own comfort zone for the needs of somebody else regardless of how tired or unhappy you are feeling at any moment. You have to be on.*

- *It's not really a job, it's your life. It's a livelihood. It encompasses every part of your life. Phone is always on. Always worried about something phone is on. It impacts on your personal life no matter how hard you try to balance it out.*

- *That we function under this burden of responsibility and if we screw up bad things will happen and we are very aware of it.*

- *People do not understand the risks that we take even emotionally when bad things happen. That kind of responsibility is very stressful, it's a good thing but it's hard. It's not just years for training and the debt that you go into but it is also the personal and emotional risks that you take.*

- *Death and dying and paperwork. That we are being bogged down by a bunch of bullshit.*

- *All of the things that happen behind the scenes, not just the exam room. And there are so many more things that we need to keep track of while we are in the exam room. Too much data that we need to put in all the right the fields, that is not always useful information but we have to do it for Meaningful Use and other quality measures. Also Patient Centered Home. All of these things need to be factored in and we need to have specific data for each of the things we are part of.*

- *One has to balance so many demands made on you from all sources. Medicine is an art not a science. It is not black or white. Lots of grays in there.*

- *They don't have the necessary experience and knowledge. The web and the media are filled with inaccurate information. Don't accept it all. It is like the world. Some is right some is not. Some people take it as gospel.*

- *Managing patients' expectations is a challenge in terms of what they are going to get from their visits. Doctors are portrayed as having all of the answers and can solve all problems. Functional and organic complaints; Problems can be sorted into these piles. Physicians in general are largely trained to treat the organic problems. Traditional medicine is poorly equipped to deal with vague pain, fatigue, headaches, and aches. There are different agendas from the patient and doctor. The doctor wants to rule out that the complaint isn't not life threatening. The patients want to feel better. The patients want to rule in and get treated. A clear mismatch which often leaves both parties dissatisfied.*

- *A doctor, a good doctor, is like a respected painter, actor, athlete, statesman. There is a combination of intellect, wit, and caring. That combination is rare.*

- *Without feeling a victim, I have a sense of being a servant. It is hard to be a doctor because of the foreign influence on the doctor-patient relationship. I have a sense especially in the hospital that I am working under bondage. The system of "accountable medicine" is creating people more interested in criticizing and attacking others that focusing onthe patients.*

- *It's not hard to be a clinician. It is difficult to be an administrator. We did not go to school learn to fill out 1,000 forms and learn every nuance of forms and new regulations. I can't bill for everything I do, the parents can't pay it.*

- *Great question. I think it is a profession when so much trust is placed on you to be benevolent, kind, patient, accurate. There is no room for a bad day. I cannot walk into a patient room without the most professional and courteous behavior. Behavioral standard has to be so high. No room for a bad day or an unprofessional moment that could haunt you for the rest of your career. That perfectionist goal is sometimes very hard.*

- *You walk in every day and you have a hard day and all day long people wait to vent to you. I am eager to hear it/have to hear it. The surgeries are fun. Being in the delivery room was fantastic. It never felt nerve wracking. I get to be part of someone's family for a little bit of time.*

- *I don't think it's hard to be a doctor. I just show up. Everything else is great. It's hard to fulfill the things that have nothing to do with being a doctor, like the business aspect and government interaction.*

- *Our educational system is so flawed in preparing doctors compared to other countries and societies. It is extremely expensive. This means investing a decade of life when friends are making money and establishing themselves financially and a career a business. Having massive student loan debt equivalent to a house mortgage or more. Yet when you start working there is no money to balance that out. I started 25 years ago. Numerous Wal-Mart's, Applebees, Targets — yet I don't recall a governor who inaugurated a medical school. The number of medical school slots has not changed but the population has doubled. 1940s post World War II it was 140 million. Nursing schools have shut down. We are focused on health care and the doctor has to comply. Regulations, mandates: OSHA JCAHO HIPAA. There is nothing that safeguards the wellbeing of healthcare workers.*

- *Trying to balance so much information and integrate information that matters for life or death. Trying to get information from people who don't want to give it to you and all in 15 minutes. Trying to balance what each patient wants. They each think that they are your only patient.*

- *Because nobody appreciates the degree of stress, thought, and time that goes into it. The sleepless nights when I am afraid for someone and worried and maybe I forgot something. It's hugely demanding with little compensation. They need to understand that it is not easy and not financially rewarding to be a primary care doctor. They should be compliant. We are telling them what is in their best interest and they don't necessarily listen.*

- *They expect perfection and expect everyone to have excellent health. So much prevention is to change wrong behaviors. There is so much that they need to do that they don't understand. But they smoke, sleep around, use drugs etc. Insurance rewards that by covering everything.*

- *Outside influences make it hard. The recertification, the exams, seeing your income decrease and expenses go up. 60 percent of our income is now expenses.*

Q: How did you balance your personal life with being a doctor?

*As one doctor interviewee said, "It's a constant struggle."

• *Always a balance. It's a constant struggle.*

• *I will let you know when I figure it out. It is difficult to balance a personal life. When I am here I feel I am guilty because I am not at home. If I am not here, I feel guilty. I have to do all things for all patients all the time. It is hard. My wife is a physician and we live close by so we tag team and juggle. We try to be there and go to all the events for the kids.*

 * *It's hard on the families and the doctors give up and miss out on a lot.*

• *Give up a lot. Working. On call. Can't just walk away. If someone is dying it affects me. I have known them for x number of years they are like extended family. Can have 10 or 15 people die. I see them more often than my parents and they depend on me. Don't want to give up –this is medicine and you have a family and a life and have an obligation to them. Don't skimp on them. Even though the patients don't think so. They have to be like part of your family. But it's hard. If I go on vacation and I'll have a patient panic – what will I do if I get sick? How dare you be away when I am sick? Every once in a while someone will say that it's good for me to recharge my battery. Or "Why are you here on Saturday?"*

• *It's very hard, especially if I am on my own. Sometimes the family becomes secondary with my own practice and trying to keep everyone happy. You try and do so much at home, it is hard, I would love to do homework and go to their games, my wife does most of it. We have two kids. It's tough, especially on your own. It's getting harder to survive on your own.*

- *I don't do well. My poor husband. The patients need me. He knows that. We have been married for many years.*

- *I don't know that I do. It's not always in balance. No such thing as balance. Some days I am a really good doctor, some days I'm a really great mom. As women we're lied to that we can have it all and we can't. I couldn't do it without a very flexible partner. He has not advanced his career to be the more accessible parent.*

- *It's been tough. You need a very understanding spouse and family. It's a lot of stress. Try very hard not to take professional life into private life. You are never on time anywhere. You are always called when you have to be somewhere. It is hard to make plans. It is hard to go away.*

- *It's hard, I need more down time. I am good at compartmentalizing.*

- *It is very difficult. It's easy to be a doctor. It is hard to have everything else. Patients are always in the back of your mind. For example, with a recent procedure. Nothing I can do to alleviate that stress.*

- *I always am a doctor. I exercise and be with my family. But I am a doctor 24/7. I am married to a physician too and that helps.*

- *HAH. I am probably like most male doctors in that the professional life had a larger importance than it should be. The younger generation does a better job. Baby boomers are workaholics and we focus on getting things done. Our kids probably saw that and rebelled so that their primary focus is creating balance. This creates tension in practice – there is a tension between the younger docs and the older ones.*

Others, like lawyers, will tell you the same thing. Not just the northeast. You will find it in Iowa.

* Some of the doctors talked about strategies and solutions for balance.

• *It takes me a long time to get rid of the mommy guilt. I do it by convincing myself that I am setting a good example for my kids. I try to isolate myself from my work when I am with my kids. I have learned to communicate more with my spouse about what I am doing and if I am brusque if he calls when I with a patient, I am not brushing them aside. I am managing that I can be with them. I have learned to tell my spouse that I will be home 90 minutes later than I will anticipate. So if I get home early it is a pleasant surprise, not a disappointment because I am late.*

• *There are days that are overwhelming. You compartmentalize and get good at it. Some patients become friends.*

• *I never had to balance my personal life. I have partners at work who always chose lifestyle over money. So we always worked really hard when we were working, but took time off too. My wife works full time. When you come home really stressed there would be a little decompression time that I need. Once I had kids I couldn't do it. Had to decompress on the car ride home.*

• *I am lucky. I have a wonderful wife. Everything is okay. She is independent. And she accepts my lifestyle.*

• *I have a large garden and I exercise. As I work more, I wonder if my personality as a doctor will change. I put up with these demanding people. I have the time.*

• *I took vacations always. I got a babysitter and went away with my wife. Most people today only go away with their kids. Once I wrote a prescription for a vacation. "Take your wife to Atlantic City for the weekend and leave the kids home," and he did. He came home and said, "Doc I am a new man". When I didn't have a nickel, I took vacations. I worked 48 weeks a year and that's it. Half the time was with the kids. I always made sure to take my wife away because she needed the break. I took each kid alone and now I do it with grandchildren. We had a motor home. I didn't just practice medicine. I was involved in medical politics, every aspect. And I involved my children.*

- *I had good childcare. You can do it. It is not as difficult. You have to have partners with you who work with you and cover for you and you do that too.*

- *Lived near my work and tried to be involved with my kids and the community.*

- *People I practiced with stayed in the office. I went home with all of my charts. I would be home and I was there. I could go into my study and work and come back out and be with the family. I came home. We were concerned about quality of life. We bought a house at the shore with which the children were involved. Quality of life for us. That helped to balance it. These things helped.*

- *I have tried to maintain a very healthy personal life throughout my career with regard to having a family and having personal interests.*

- *In this practice, and the reason we have survived, we do feel that you have a personal life. I am home by 6 or 7 if not on call, or even on call; it's not so bad. It's one weekend a month to work. We have more doctors for the same amount of work as other practices so we can do this. We are all on our first marriages, everyone, and no one has left the practice. It's a lot of work but still but my kids saw me.*

- *It helps to have a family. When I started on this whole project I had two little boys and I was pre-med. Then in my last year of medical school I had my daughter. That was hard; I had to sleep at the hospital when I was a resident and I had to leave a little baby. I have a supportive spouse. He made it easy. My kids are healthy kids who were cooperative with my need to study. I found a job as an employed physician. The person who owns it and the others are mothers and there is a lot of flex. I take off sometimes to see my granddaughter. I have a good schedule.*

- *I didn't work full time when my kids were younger, I worked part time. I have a supportive family and a good partner who makes me laugh.*

- *I have it pretty easy. It has not been difficult.*

- *There is often a back and forth because the same qualities that make you a good doctor and husband and father – the skills to listen to kids with empathy – are the same as with the patients. Same problem solving skills. They universally impact the other sphere. All of my patients have my cell phone and my email. I believe that being available is an essential part of the doctor-patient relationship. Only two have abused it.*

- *I try and turn it off at home. At home I want to be dad and husband, not doctor.*

- *I am blessed with a wonderful wife and children and I am very happy. And besides being a doctor I have a full family life.*

- *I am very blessed. I have great family support.*

- *You compartmentalize it. Feel sympathy and empathy and then move on.*

- *With a group you can take more time off. Sole practitioners are less common today. Did not feel that much interference any more than any other business. Time becomes more intensive sometimes.*

- *Balance. I compartmentalize it. I garden. I have hobbies. I don't bring it home.*

- *I work close to home. I try to limit my hours in the evening.*

- *I reinvented my career and requirements during the different stages of my children's lives when their needs were different to be available to them and not have someone else raise them, so that I could be there myself and feel fulfilled as a mother and in my career.*

- *You have to be prepared to sacrifice a lot of personal life. I hardly remember a school game or event without being interrupted with pages by pharmacies, patients, other doctors. Making sure I stop and have dinner with my kids, I look at their homework and then do more work.*

- *I try to keep things as separate as I can for my patients sake and my family.*

- *Because of my spouse. I have friends and I have a social life. I travel. We are foodies. We explore. My daughters are sweeties.*

Q: How did you/do you handle all of the feelings that go along with being a doctor?

* It's a challenge.

- *I haven't figured it out. Sometimes family has to take the brunt of it. It isn't fair to them.*

- *With practice I felt that I did it well.*

- *I don't know the answer. I just handle it. It is a big responsibility and you just do it. This is why it is so hard to take care of friends.*

- *This is true of any professional. You can't do something unless you really enjoy it, this is my advice to anyone who is choosing a career. Choose one that you can do for the rest of your life, I enjoy what I do. There are good days and bad days.*

- *There are a lot of feelings. Joy, anger. I just deal with it. You do what you have to do and move on. You are supposed to compartmentalize. I am not good at it.*

- *As well as I can.*

- *I don't know. Just trudge along and do the best you can and have fun along the way and laugh. All you can do is be the best that you can be.*

- *I was afraid of becoming a doctor, that it would eat up all of my time and I would never have fun again. I was afraid I would make a mistake and kill someone. I was afraid to watch the early medical shows. I needed to put myself through the fire. I was rebellious.*

- *I found out that I was quite good. Do I divorce myself from the intense reactions? I found that I could deal with it. I would come home from nights on call. I was literally baptized in human suffering. I realized that I needed to do that. I found out that I was a good clinician. I had been well trained in spite of myself.*

- *I cry.*

- *I wish I knew. Sometimes it is depressing. No sounding board to talk to. People don't understand.*

- *I try and compartmentalize it so that I don't bring my concerns about my patients home when I am interacting with my children and my wife and vise versa. But it is hard to always compartmentalize because there are a lot of issues that patients have and I do spend time following up on evenings and weekends and calling patients back and following up test results regardless of if I am on call or not. It's fine. It is my responsibility but it leads to the sense that you are almost never off. As you do it more over time you learn to balance it more and better.*

- *We become a little inured. We can take it. Death and sadness don't horrify me as they used to do. It's all part of the cycle of life. It is what it is. There is a lot that we can do sometimes there is nothing we can.*

- *I take patients personally and can't be cold. I try and treat them as my own children. I want the best for both. At times when I feel that someone can do it better or add something, I will enlist them and help steer the patient to get the best result rather than not share.*

- *It's a learning process. There are things that happen every day that bring you back to reexamining it. If you are not someone who constantly reexamines yourself you cannot survive in this field.*

- *Besides burying them? Not a lot of time to process them. You are really on 24/7 whether you have to pee, poop, have sex, shower, or eat, there is always someone who needs you. You have to value yourself and know what your needs are. You are the only one who will meet them.*

* Support from family and friends is helpful.

- *I just handle it. You do not have a lot of choice. Try not to get too upset about things although that never works completely. Sometimes if something really upsets me I call one of my partners as a pressure balance and just complain. It's not complaining to commiserate and share. A lot of times that is my best way to de-stress from work. My wife cares more about me but I do not have the shared experiences with her.*

- *My husband is a doctor and he gets it. We have three kids. They get it that the phone rings a lot. It's not all about them. There are other people in the world.*

- *I have a good marriage. My kids are great. My wife is the greatest. My brother and I are the best, real supportive.*

- *Process of going through all of the issues of being a physician by reaching out to my friend who is my partner for 32 years. We are like brothers; we are able to share mistakes, difficult patients and emotional pain and work it through. Also home. Wife. Children.*

- *I just handle it. My wife is a good sounding board. Sometimes it's not easy. Sometimes I get down.*

- *I talk to other doctors and friends and my husband.*

- *I am blessed to have an excellent practice with nice patients and I don't feel particularly stressed. Satisfying career, I like the people I work with and I like what I do.*

- *You train yourself to be numb.*

- *Through my personal faith.*

- *I talk to other people who take care of patients who are as sick as mine and commiserate about how it was so hard. I linger in the office at night until I can get someone to talk to. It adds to my spouse's stress level.*

Q: What did you need that you didn't have?

*Some of the doctor interviewees don't report any unmet needs.

- *I feel that I was prepared.*

- *I can't think of anything.*

- *I had a good support system. I was lucky.*

* The unmet needs are all related to business, feelings, and clinical skills. It's the same themes.

- *I need a winning lottery ticket, so that I can do it without the stresses of running a business.*

- *A life. You spend most of your 20s in school and most of our friends are going on vacation and partying. We miss out of all of it. Getting married and having kids like a side event. Not getting to enjoy it as much as other professionals. Working long hours, have to work your way up all along the way. Student. Resident. Fellowship, practice. It's a long up and down and before you know it you are in your 30s and half your life is over. I had a lot. My father worked hard did a lot of different things. So, I learned to work hard. I worked hard, I saw my dad do it. I wanted to have a better life. Now, paperwork and changes are happening in healthcare that are going to affect all of us. Accountable Care Organizations hospitals are buying practices and then you lose those referrals if physicians become part of that group and have their own specialist. It will be tough to survive on your own.*

- *My parents. They died when I was too young.*

- *A financial background.*

- *Better partners.*

- *I didn't have any of the stuff we do for the residents now.*

For example, if a kid dies. You had to deal with the feelings on your own. We do a lot more for our trainees.

- *I was naïve and didn't have what my partner did for me. Being with him gave me legitimacy. He was my partner and we were great friends. I thanked him. It carried me in my earlier years. So proud to be his partner. There were five of us. Once a month we had a dinner together. It was really fun. It was wonderful we got along so well, we helped each other out. This is what the public needs to understand. We doctors are always constantly learning.*

- *Maybe people in solo practice didn't have a partner. But I had coverage every other night and weekend.*

- *I wish I had a little better business acumen. I wish I had a couple of better partners. I wish I had better rates of reimbursement. Otherwise I do not sit here and complain. We have been hit with forces of medical change, so we have learned how to mutate like viruses to survive. We may have the capacity to do that. I can hire staff and see more patients.*

- *A million dollars. More free time.*

- *Time. And all of the things that I need to take care of and document. I would like more time to read medical journals and go to conferences.*

- *Time.*

- *There is one thing. I wish I had been just a little bit smarter. Maybe I could have saved a few more people. I could have found the answer a little sooner.*

- *Wisdom.*

- *I was raised to be a very trusting person. I still have a certain naiveté and trust that may not sure it works in my favor. It is very rare to find someone you can really trust. You need some skepticism.*

- *Some training with billing, administration. It has been a horrendous uphill learning experience. A block box. Wish I had been taught. The business of medicine. Cannot survive without it. All trial and error.*

- *Some training in how to deal with the stress of insurance, legal, deal with all the feelings.*

- *Capitated medicine has transformed into a business with big massive government and insurance. The heath care worker is a pawn in that process and you have to hang on for dear life. I had fantasies about starting a diabetes campus in a friendly environment. It needs capital investment to hire dieticians, nurses, counselors. Hospitals will build a parking lot of a $5 million machine. We lose the element of the human person, which is the most important one. When it comes to developing the heath care worker, you are on your own. So many barriers for someone who wants to do something and being the best you can be. You are left to your own to fight it. No one asks the doctors how we feel.*

- *A mentoring physician. I did not have a lot support. There was a lot of competition. Not an infrastructure of support.*

- *Financial recognition for working my ass off all of these years. Primary care physicians don't make a lot of money. There have been weeks where I paid my staff, paid their 401K's and paid all of my bills but didn't pay myself.*

CHAPTER 3

THE PATIENTS

What is it/was it like working with patients?

* Very much like what was described in most of the doctor books in the References section at the end of this book, most of the interviewees found working with patients to be a positive experience. As one of my interviewees said, "It is why I do what I do."

• *That's great. I like it.*

• *Love it. Still love it. I know my patients in and out. I have taken care of three generations. I know about their job and kids. That is what is really fun. My patients know the names of my children and my wife works in my office. Pictures of my grandson in my office. They stop in at our shore home. They are part of our personal life. We get intruded up on sometimes, but I really like my patients.*

• *When I am in the room and the door is closed, I am happy. I can be there with the patients and I can help them. This is why I went into medicine. Sometime they need something and I want to help them and help them be better people. Then I open the door and all the other crap hits. When I have been with them and established a relationship it is great. Sometime patients think that I am only in it for the money and I am in it for myself.*

• *It's wonderful. I love patients. It is why I do what I do.*

• *It's fun. I get to be close to them immediately because of their trust in me. I don't see the walls that they put up to the rest of the world; they include me with everything that goes on in their life. Usually.*

- *For me it's just my job, as a family doc. I enjoy learning things like what jobs they have and I am interested in them as people. I have fabulous artists.*

- *I went into my subspecialty to take care of families in a long term way and help them take care of their diseases over the long term and have a relationship with them.*

- *I look at suffering as God is suffering. I treat my patients as if I am loving God through them. It is sacred and you do your best.*

- *Easy. Not too many patients that have made life impossible.*

- *It's fine.*

- *I love it. They all have stories and I love listening to their stories.*

- *It's great.*

- *I like my patients. I like 95% of them. They come in and talk to me and I get paid.*

- *This is the best part of medicine. You get to know them as humans. Who they are, what kind of work to they do, fears and hopes, and try to be the steward of their health.*

- *I love it. I am a coach, not a provider.*

- *Like a daily therapy session. I share a bit of my personal life and I get ideas and support. It keeps me going.*

* Working with patients is clinically interesting.
- *It is interesting. Every patient is different. They have different stories, strengths and weaknesses.*

- *It is great. It is a learning experience.*

- *It's interesting because you have people from different backgrounds. Everyone brings something else to the table. Some people want to keep it superficial. Some want to tell you about their families. For the most part people give respect and trust your judgment.*

- *This is what I like. Everyone is different. You can have the same diagnosis in 10 patients and it is like having 10 different patients.*

* Being a doctor does have its negatives, even if it's mostly positive. The negatives could be related to business or feelings, or clinical issues.

- *Some of them have a sense of humor. I have a great staff. It's a privilege to be let into their lives and to work with them. Sometimes it's sad.*

- *I really enjoy my encounter with them. I like talking with them. Sometimes it is difficult. In the ER the behaviorally disturbed patients were really difficult. One guy was discharged by the psychiatrist and he killed himself.*

- *Some people are shits and don't deserve you and some people are exceptionally nice. Most people appreciate you and some people don't and they make you hate them too.*

- *For the most part working with patients is joyful, see a patient for the first time. It takes time to develop a relationship. The patients I have been seeing for years are wonderful. Talk about medical and other stuff and that is what keeps me going. I still enjoy dealing with people in general not just a doc to patients all the time. But we have our limits in the relationships. But some of them are my friends. People I would have never have met otherwise. For the most part people do appreciate it. There is a trend over the last 5 to10 years. I feel like patients come to a physician to either leave with a medicine or have a specific answer as to why they are the way they are and they want an easy solution. I don't see the accountability and people saying I have to eat better,* stop smoking and exercise. The onus is on us to do everything. There is pressure on us to do things that we cannot do. How can we make them do things? No accountability. If I didn't document well and something happens, it could be a real problem. Sometimes you are in a rush on the phone, in the hospital and shopping and tell them what to do and you can't document everything. So busy. If there is a bad outcome. No matter how unaccountable the patient is for their own health they will blame the physicians 9 out of 10 times. I have patients who are so meticulous and I have the opposite what is going on with them. You have to spoon feed them everything and they still don't do it. Need different hats for different personalitiesto get into their heads to make a difference. You can't document that in notes. I can't document a relationship in writing. How I was telling them and how I tried to get through to them is not in my notes. I feel like doctors are getting a bad rap. The few are in it for the many. People go out in the middle of the night and will call patients and it doesn't get recognized. Compare to physicians who don't care. I don't think that good physicians get recognized and get lumped in with the bad ones. The ones who are trying to do better. Impossible to measure. You can't know. No measure of how many people I have prevented from serious illness. No way to measure that. The only way to know is to follow him around. My patients are fragile and serious and one little thing sends them to the ICU. I don't get paid for seeing some of the patients. I went to the hospital to see a patient who I had already seen that day. I will not get paid.

- I loved working with my patients; 95% of my patients were wonderful people who I became close with. A 10% are difficult with everyone. They make it like you cringe but you still have to work with them.

- *The whole point of clinical medicine is to work with patients. So if you don't like that you are in the wrong field. Most good doctors want to please their patients by making them feel better. I don't like conformation and conflict though.*

- *I find it my greatest joy except when they try to take advantage of me. When they understand me and when they think that I understand them, they really listen to me.*

- *I like working with patients. That is what I am here for. Some are more difficult than others. Some need more time. In the end it evens out.*

- *Not always on your game. No one is. There are some hours or days of just going through the motions. When you are really on the game, it's really nice. I get to have 20 meaningful conversations a day. People are appreciative and say thank you. Some of these people make an impact. Others I don't think that I am making an impact, but they do.*

- *I love the interaction. Typically it is a very enjoyable experience. We have parents too and I like it. There are negative experiences with some parents but generally speaking parents want the best for their kids. It is negative to have to run after them to come back.*

- *I enjoy the patients. Even the pains in the asses. Very few patients I have hated. I like the patients.*

* In one interview, the concern about finances came up early. More on this topic later.

- *There is something that has changed a bit in becoming a doctor that I didn't have to deal with. Incredible student loans. It is incredible impact. It is a deterrent. You could go to Wall Street or be an attorney. You can't pay them back. It impacts who decided to be a doctor.*

Q: Please tell me your thoughts on the doctor-patient relationship. Does it matter? If so, why?

* Research has shown that the doctor patient relationship is a key part, quite possibly the most important part, of healthcare. Dr. Bonnie Svastad and colleagues demonstrated that it impacts compliance. Later studies — such as by Dr. Alexander and colleagues, and the Nuance Foundation — confirm the importance of the relationship for patient health outcomes.

* One of the doctor interviewees for this book made the important connection that the destruction of the doctor-patient relationship by insurance companies actually raises the cost of healthcare because it affects compliance. A prime example of the importance of the relationship for health outcomes was given by one of my interviewees. "For example, with a blood transfusion, the hospitalist couldn't get a patient to do it," one doctor said. "His primary care MD called and got him to agree to it in a few minutes."

* No disagreement here in these interviews about the importance of the doctor-patient relationship. As one of the doctor interviewees said, "It is everything. We are losing it." As another one said, "With a strong relationship your voice will be in their heads at home." And as one doctor interviewee stated, "It matters the most because a good relationship means compliance and compliance means better outcomes which costs less."

• *It's important. I do primary care, so you have to have that relationship. They always harp on compliance. How do you get the patients to comply? You have to have a relationship to care and be interested in them and then they will follow what you say to do. It has to be this way so that the patient will follow your care and keep coming back and asking for your help when they need it. If you have no interest or act like a robot they won't comply.*

- *Intimate. It matters to the extreme. It is what makes people better more often than medication.*

- *Bonding.*

- *That's where it is and where it all starts. It's almost everything. It matters. If the relationship is good it opens everything up to taking good care of somebody. The person will listen to your recommendations because they trust you. If it's not a good relationship they may not listen because of that, i.e. diet or smoking or not getting a stress test. On the negative end I have these nervous patients who won't do anything without me. I have to call them before they agree to do anything that the specialist is recommending. It gets frustrating that is keeping me there later. Biopsy the breast mass or get the colonoscopy. I have to beg. Don't wait two weeks. Seven days a week and we are open 'til 9 most days. Don't wait two weeks for me. There are other doctors to see besides me. Don't leave your strep untreated while waiting. Don't love them. Don't hate them. Just treat them.*

- *Yes, they need that trust to come to you. You need someone to be focused and help you. Even if they go to Sloane, they call me. The trust factor. I think that it helps them. No question that it is important and it is good for their health.*

- *It's important. It has to be earned and they have to see that you really care. It makes a significant difference to help them with the right treatment. They trust you to give them the right treatment or to be honest that you don't know.*

- *I already touched on it. It matters. It is essential. If you don't have it you will misdiagnose and not give them the proper care. If you don't like it get out. If you don't like your doctor get another one, have a good fit. If you want someone to tell you what to do you find someone who will do that. It definitely matters. You cannot get good patient care without it.*

- *It is critical. They tell me such stories if they don't open up to me. I can help them more when they tell me what they are worried about like a headache and a brain tumor. I have patients who don't tell me that they drink until they get in trouble. I thought that I had a relationship. I feel bad for them. They didn't tell me so that I could intervene. One patient died.*

- *Important to diagnosis, as the patient feels free to discuss with the doctor. The more you know about the patient, work, and family.*

- *Enormously matters. Trust issues. I let my guard down and talk about my inadequacies easily. That helps too.*

- *The doctor-patient relationship takes what we do out of the dimension of strictly delivering a service. Sometimes I can do an exam relatively quickly and spend the rest of the time talking about children, bereavement, interests. We have developed a relationship over the years and we are interested in each other's lives to the degree that they intersect and we can share that. I have learned more about how people cope with loss than almost anything else, because I have found that people were coming in coping with loss and I did not want to sit there and be awkward and change the subject, I wanted to learn to explore being of comfort and assistance. I had to learn how to speak of these things and I had known nothing about it beforehand. I let patients sit and cry in my office and cry for as long as they need to about things that have nothing to do with their exam because that particular day they needed to come to someone's office and cry. The exam was sort of a bonus.*

- *It matters a lot. Have to have trust. If not it is done. They have to trust you and you have to trust them or the relationship is sunk. It's not that different from my car guy. I don't have the fund of knowledge about cars. The relationship matters a lot. I discussed it once with a hospitalist. They just know the patients when they come in. There is no relationship. They see them once. For example, with a blood transfusion, he couldn't get a patient to do it. His primary care MD called and got him to agree to it in a few minutes.*

- *A matter of trust. If the patient feels that his or her welfare is my primary concern. Without that trust nothing works.*

- *Pearl of wisdom. In medical school, I came across an old family doc. He said, "Don't try to be a doctor for every patient. Be the doctor you want to be, and the patients will self select."*

- *It is everything and it's why they keep coming back. We are in a unique position to make a difference. I get an opportunity to intervene. The spouses will often say you tell him. He will listen to you. They say having a good relationship avoids malpractice suits. Sometimes.*

- *It definitely matters in the kind of work that I do. So much of primary care is not just the science. If you have a good relationship it helps you do your job better. You can uncover things that you need to make the diagnosis. A lot of physical symptoms are related to emotional life and history. If someone is not comfortable telling you, you can miss a large piece of the puzzle.*

- *It's the most important thing if the patient can't trust you.*

- *It matters the most because a good relationship means compliance and compliance means better outcomes which costs less.*

- *Supremely sacred and never to be violated. I can't even discuss my patients with my wife.*

- *It matters tremendously. It is not a placebo. The patient being heard in a private way that does not have to leave the room has a healing effect. It is such a privilege. Enriches my life and healing for the patient. Nothing is more precious. I am constantly striving to preserve. It is endangered.*

- *I love it. I'm in a unique position. Can help patients change things they could not change before. Absolutely. The patients have usually left a doctor that they didn't have a good relationship with.*

- *Yes it matters. Not with every patient. Some patients come in and I could be a machine. All they want is to feel better or whatever their agenda is. But there are a lot of patients and there is a real relationship. They ask how I am etc. A patient where I practiced before was sorry that I was coming back to New Jersey. He was looking forward to growing old with me. As I have gotten older I have gotten better at sharing parts of my life with them. I am not a robot.*

- *I don't socialize with my patients. They can count on me to tell them the truth. I have no economic incentives so I tell them the best thing to do. No surgi-center, no drug companies. I don't own x-ray equipment.*

- *Yes it is very important. Have to enlist the patient if you want them to do well. I enjoy that. With both parents and patients. I don't wear a white jacket. The white jackets make the babies cry. I dress eclectic. I share with my 15-year-old daughter. Younger and funky. It helps them relax.*

* The doctor patient relationship has changed, and not for the better. Much of this change is attributed to insurance problems.

• *The doctor-patient relationship has changed. The best relationships are the older patients who grew up when a doctor was respected. They are grateful and there is a certain level of respect there. I try and give them respect too. I rarely call them by their first name. It doesn't bother me so much anymore when they do it to me.*

• *It is everything. We are losing it. This is not much not just with me and with the referring physicians. Some of the patients don't like their other physicians some physicians cannot take the time with their patients. You have to create a relationship you have to take time to do it. It helps their outcomes and your satisfaction. It's everything. It is the most important thing about how a patient does. You have to have it to get them to buy in and do it for themselves. With a strong relationship your voice will be in their heads at home.*

• *That is the problem now. The relationship has been chipped away. They try and take it away. And some doctors now are blind like robots. It's easier. If you invest in them, they switch anyway. Everyone is against you. So you pull back and withdraw. You do not want to be a target and getting attacked. It hurts when you are being attacked. Meanwhile when you get sick who is taking care of you? Who calls your insurance to advocate for you? The patients are so entitled. They expect you to do it. They yell if it's not fast enough. The patient has a lot to do with the relationship and they are like spoiled brats. They go online and go to the insurance companies. They are taking everything, even self esteem, away from the doctor.*

- *We had an ethics module in medical school. Important not to be paternalistic. Give full disclosure and give all options. Others don't do it. I am there to access and give information to make a good decision that works for their own family. Medical training now is all shift work. For me it's not. My patients are my patients 24 hours a day. Even on the weekends. They are my responsibility. Shift work is a great way for bad things to happen. With the shift work no one will know what is going on with us.*

- *I think that it really matters, we are losing it. Medicine is becoming corporate. Big groups and number crunching and new hospitalists. They don't know the person. When I go into a hospital room I know that patient like the back of my hand. I know their meds and tests. It is being lost.*

- *Sometimes our MD's feel angry and frustrated. It's not personal. They are not bad medical people. But there is often a disconnect on multiple levels. They do care so much about their patients.*

- *It's changing. People are getting in the way. It's hard to develop a relationship if you know it could be gone in a moment if their insurance changes.*

- *A lot. Everybody has their nose in it. Everyone has their nose in it and have no idea what they are talking about. Forms, regulations, and rules. They screw it up.*

- *The doctor-patient relationship is a closed entity system and anything that affects the doctor will affect the patients. Because of the third-party pressure, the relationship has become dry and aloof. "Cortical". I want a relationship that includes the heart and the mind. The increasing litigation and the internet have contributed to producing patients that see the doctor like a product to be consumed or something to be taking profit from with lawsuits.*

- *It matters, I think. I don't think that every doctor today feels the same way. There are a lot of doctors for whom, because of what is happening with reimbursement going down and practice expenses constantly going up, the only way to be financially viable is to increase volume. Spend less time with the patient to increase hours which also increases overhead. So the best thing is to see more patients. This is more profitable. The main thing that fosters the doctor-patient relationship is the time that you send talking and listening. That will suffer. Not every patient is interested in the relationship.*

- *It has really been stressed over the past five to ten years because of billing and reimbursement issues. I am very acutely aware of the financial stresses on families today. Explanation of benefits statements are not easy to read and understandable. When I call my own company to find out why something was not medically necessary, i.e. a melanoma. How can a procedure recommended by a doctor be deemed medically unnecessary? It should not even exist.*

- *It is most important. There are lots of intrusions from third-party people. Faxing notes on the patients to Horizon for a subtracting agency for another third party who codes and reviews. All of that so that the end of the day they can send you $11 for the visit but they have already come down on the fee. Yet they have generated so many levels of intrusions and cost for that one visit. It comes out of the premiums the patients pay to hire those armies of reviewers who are shadowing every whisper that the patient makes.*

- *It's key. If it's not there the patient won't trust you and take your advice. It's the key to being a successful physician.*

- *The doctor-patient relationship is one of the most intimate relationships that exists. People who are literally stripped naked both psychologically and physically, and what is being lost here is that relationship. A wedge is being driven in there. Healthcare is derivative of the culture from which it springs. Everyone wants for free.*

- *Very important, obviously. It is important to be respectful of the patients and families for all comers. The majority of patients are very respectful. Important to maintai patient confidentiality.*

Q: PLEASE TELL ME ABOUT YOUR MOST DIFFICULT PATIENTS.

* Some difficulties are clinical. Similar patient situations are described in some of the doctor books, but it seems that they have become more frequent and hard to manage.

- *I have a patient in my practice who is genuinely sick. She has a very rare medical condition with bizarre and somatic unrelated complaints. She is anxious and controlling. She goes from one specialist to another. It's not enough for her to explain her symptoms. Her life is spent in perpetual search for a solution. She is not crazy. She has a serious medical illness, but it is not curable and she compounds the problem by interacting with the medical system.*

- *Those with bad diseases. Difficult problems, not difficult people.*

* Patients who are abusive, ungrateful, manipulative, or entitled are difficult.

- *Drug addicts. Sneaky. They prey on a person like me because I am sympathetic.*

- *Those who think that I am super rich and can afford to give anything to them for free.*

- *I had to call the police one time. The patient wouldn't stop screaming. 99.99% are great. If I get pissed off I tell them there are 100 doctors in this town. Pick one.*

- *Those who are ungrateful.*

- *The ones who manipulative patients and those who want pain medicines. Those can be difficult. Non-compliant patients. Come for one visit and expect me to handle everything else by phone and don't want to pay or pay co-pays. I try to keep them happy. I used to wait things but I don't do it now. Different personalities. I see patients from the area's indigent populations. Underserved areas. They are challenging. They are angry, mad at the world. They come in here and it is hard to get them to do anything. Demanding patients. These are the patients who are willing to sue. Did your best and not able to document all of these interactions. It's always in the back of your head. You have to be careful, can't let it drive how you practice but it is hard. Try to help people who don't help themselves.*

- *Some people just want to take up a lot of time. Sometimes I am afraid of being sued. I don't worry as much now. I am not a specialist. They want to monopolize the time.*

- *The patient who is abusive to the staff. Or they say that they want to change and they don't. It's hard to watch them get less and less healthy over the years.*

* Some are related to negative patient behavior, and these are often the most difficult situations. For example, one doctor interviewee said, "Sometimes people aren't nice." It's not always a clinical problem. "Not the most intractable medical problems. The ones who are angry at the world."

- *Passive aggressive, not involved in self care.*

- *In my specialty we have some very serious illnesses. I took care of an immigrant seven or eight years ago. Serious involvement and we thought he would die. A poor man on Medicaid. I worked hard to make him feel better. He survived and is healthy. This whole family comes and brings food, meals, gifts, and took us out for dinner. It was a challenging case. It is the American dream. He made a plaque to honor me. On the other hand I have a patient who is a professional who is so annoying. He became my patient and fights me about everything. He has limited knowledge. The office visits are confrontational. I yell at him.*

- *Who have the least wrong with them.*

- *I have a list of about 10. Multiple Personality Disorder. Splitting. Dissociative Identity Disorder. A couple of them. A mom who killed herself. She was bi-polar. That was awful. A couple of kids shot themselves. Drug addict deaths. The worst patients are four relationship squares. Lovely family with a minor problem. The lovely family who has a child who is seriously ill don't mind taking care of them, they work with, you are grateful. The difficult people who drive anyone crazy and they try to control everything and the kid is really sick. The worst is the difficult family with a minor problem; they will drive you crazy. Another kid is dying and their Jello is not right and they yell at the nurse and the resident. Only one or a few times I had to walk away. I had to fire patients in practice. A family accused me of scratching the baby, so I said, "So find another doctor." I have never been sued.*

- *There are two types. My narcotic patients and the demanding patients. They think that they are the only patient in the world. Passive aggressive. Just call me and let me know what went wrong so that I can try and fix it.*

- *Sued me or refused to take responsibility for themselves. Constantly on the phone or making appointments with questions any grandmother could answer.*

- *Drug addicts. Borderlines. The ones who come cursing their last doctor. You are next.*

- *Those with borderline personality disorder.*

- *Not the most intractable medical problems. The ones who are angry at the world, at medicine, at their families. They are angry and determined to come in and find fault with whatever we do regardless of what it is.*

- *Have personality issues. Different kinds of difficult. I am uncomfortable and I can't figure out what is wrong. It is not the patient's fault. Then there are people who are very demanding, unfriendly, negative. Depressed patients are often difficult even though I understand. The outright crazies are difficult but less so. The schizophrenics were fine. Sociopaths, you can't treat them. They were miserable. Can't treat them. If you want to fight with them, you can't get anywhere. They don't want to listen and they are arguing. Very negative patients. Cognitive problems and they are sadder. They are sad but not contentious. The nurses spend a lot of them on the phone with them. It's sad. Hard to watch. I have known some of them have had their cognitive decline and I have watched them. Not always proud of how*

I handle it. Every once in a while someone will set you off and you have to control yourself. People want things that as a specialist I don't do. I do not have the full knowledge base for these other fields.

- *I don't have anyone in mind, so I guess that's good. I don't do hospital medicine anymore but this was in the beginning. She had a medical issue but also borderline personality disorder and I kept being pulled in and I didn't know what to do about it. And then there was one more who clearly had very severe OCD. She couldn't even come to the office without putting everyone through all of her allergies, etc.*

- *Needy. You come out of the exam room sucked dry. Not bad people. Passive aggressively demanding.*

- *Two categories: those with medical problems and serious behavioral categories. Most difficult in the behavioral was when the patents disagreed, for example on how to raise the children. So many meetings trying to find common ground.*

- *I am a little different than other doctors. Mine are the most challenging and I don't mind them. It is nice when something is straightforward, but when you have a patient with a lot of anxiety and denial and PTSD, who have a lot of functional disease and have difficulty seeing the relationship between somatic and psychological issues. Hard to get through it but when you do it is gratifying. The most difficult ones are the ones who only want to talk and do not want to listen. A powerful commitment to a preconceived agenda and you can't sway them until you ask why they are here.*

- *They usually present with a problem that has been self-diagnosed via the internet. Need to tell the patient that they aren't wrong but they may not be right.*

* Sometimes the difficulty has more to do with family members of the patient.

• *Two types of difficulty. The patient who is extremely sick and takes an enormous amount of time in giving them the right treatment. Then where is the patient who is easier to treat but the family is dysfunctional and so it is hard to negotiate their care. They don't know me. They have guilt, anger, frustrations related to their family members. Those are the hardest.*

• *More and more I don't have difficult patients, I have difficult families. I have older patients with a great relationship and then they get sick in the hospital and the family members come out of the woodwork and I have no relationship and they have no relationship and I have to work on winning them over. The non- compliant patients. I treat opiate addictions and they are difficult and manipulative. They can also be so rewarding. Getting them off the addiction and see how their lives have changed.*

• *The patients are not difficult. It's the family members that can't accept what is going on. Especially with older people and ambivalent feelings and can't write up a DNR. Completely unrealistic. Or call me all the time for not valid feelings and they don't want to come in and see me. They don't want to come in and see me and pay me. Patients who don't understand that I am entitled to make money, not a huge amount, or fill out six forms for free. Not possible. When I go home at 9 at night I don't want to fill out forms. Most of them are nice. Have to understand where they are coming from. It's amazing how well they deal. They are getting old and they don't feel good, they have pain all over their body but they tough it out.*

- *There's all sorts of patients. I don't know what is going on, so I am not making the right diagnosis. Patients are angry at me and can be demanding. I am frustrated that they are not feeling well and I for whatever reason I am not helping them.*

- *Two types. The ones who won't come back and say on the phone everything is fine, but you don't know. It's frustrating. Over attentive parents looking for too much. It s more psychological. My associate handles some of these issues. I have learned a lot from him. Practice changes. I have some DYFS patients. I almost sent the cops out looking for them the other day. He's in foster care.*

* Non-compliance makes it difficult to care for patients. Ultimately this affects health outcomes. These responses of these doctor interviewees support the established research, discussed earlier.

- *The non-compliant patients.*

- *I would say that the most difficult patients are the ones that have difficulty following medical instructions with medications, lifestyle cessation, smoke. Patients with heart attacks, stents, who still smoke. It's like committing suicide every day. Clog up your body. Ignoring near and dear ones.*

- *Those who do not take care of themselves. And they are headed towards complications and you are not able to convey that importance. And those who are disrespectful to our staff. They are very caring and compassionate and respectful and we expect the patients to be respectful. If they have complaints of grievances they need to approach it with a more civilized manner.*

- *It's not the medical issues. It's their personalities that are difficult. It's the inability to be truthful and not cover up their shortcomings. Non-compliance. We handle it with patience, with yelling and sometimes with begging. I have been known to get on my knees and beg and it doesn't work usually.*

- *We always talk about patient compliance. It is difficult when, for example with diabetes, but they are not paying attention to complying. They may not understand the significance, be in denial, or because it is hard to do. Tough and challenging scenarios. I like the challenge, so it is okay. It is hard because I know that they are increasing their potential for long term negative outcomes. We try and work with them and help them understand, get their perspective, involve the family members. For children, try and empower the teenagers to take control.*

- *This was a child with severe chronic illness and my treatment recommendations were not being followed. The outcome was not good.*

- *A recent patient who didn't want surgery. She almost died. I tried to compromise until the last minute.*

- *The ones who may have unhealthy lifestyle and want to change, but for various reasons cannot. When my pep talks fails, it can be hard on the patient and me just to find a middle ground. Sometimes it's really hard to find ways to be constructive. Or if there is not a good treatment. Providing support when there is no treatment and trying to keep the patent in the driver's seat in his or her life. The Nature of Suffering (book by Dr. E. Cassell). Not just the physical suffering, but the loss of control over your life. But you can help provide that to the patient and the family.*

- *Borderlines. We talked about one example. The people who don't want to listen. Or have had difficult patients when they have an agenda which doesn't match mine, like not wanting to go to work. I am pretty lenient, but… one patient wanted a note from two months ago. Mostly when they don't listen. To an extreme. Most patients don't listen.*

Q: WHAT MADE THIS/THESE PATIENTS SO DIFFICULT?

*Again, entitlement is difficult.

• *More difficult. More demanding. It's our culture, instant gratification. That's just not the way medicine works. It's a different animal.*

• *They have no perspective and have no idea what it means to have a child with a real problem or a hard life or real pain or real hardship. The majority of people don't want to change their lifestyle. In fellowship, our chairman was dealing with people complaining about the food when they were there for a minor problem. He would move them in with a sick child and within 24 hours there was no more complaining.*

• *Their sense of entitlement.*

• *The "You owe me" mentality.*

* Mental health problems often cause difficulties. More on mental health aspects of healthcare later in this chapter.

• *They are not nice. They are not honest with themselves. There is always a world around them that is to blame.*

• *Their inborn inabilities to handle problems themselves. They should know. Or refer to someone else if it is something beyond what I can handle – medical or psychologists or psychiatrists if it was based in such problems.*

• *Them trying to put things in the way of medical issues in order to get care that they need that has nothing to do with medical issues. Confusing to separate physical and emotional problems. I probably see equal amounts of each. Where I had to say "I won't take care of you."*

Misc
- *Do you get less patient as you get older or more patient? Yes and no. There are pussy cats and bears patients.*

Q: How did you handle it?

* One strategy is to persist. Another is to accept that nothing can really be done.

- *Encourage them.*

- *I say the same thing again and again. Hard for them to understand or motivate themselves. I believe that as physicians if we say the same thing again and again one day they will listen to what trying to say.*

- *I handle it by empathizing with their not follow up. I am not perfect and so we moved on and try and do better. People who walk in and curse and scream, they can't curse at my staff. They are nice to me and the staff doesn't get that. My staff wants me to see something. Our phone conversations are taped. They say they weren't rude to the staff. We have video cameras.*

- *By not being angry. Not being judgmental and listening to what they want to do and present the options and let people know here is no right or wrong answer and you will work with them for the better cause for their relative.*

- *Usually I just keep trying and trying and trying and handle it over and over again.*

- *As much TLC as you can.*

- *Gently. I try and take her and see things from her perspective and I have a hard time because she is so different from me and I can't get into her crazy world. I felt guilty that I am unable to help her in an objective sort of way.*

- *With courtesy and seeing them as beggars and with compassion.*

- *They have their own personal struggles and issues.*

* There are often attempts to educate the patient or to set limits. If that attempt fails, sometimes it is suggested that the patients go elsewhere for their care.

- *Yoga. I try to not get caught in their upward spiral. Be calm. And I set very clear boundaries. If you don't want to do it, don't come back. No one has ever talked to them. I try not to get caught in their crazy. I feel pretty good at it.*

- *We throw people out of our practice. If they are nice to me but not my staff, we throw them out. Life is too short to deal with nasty people.*

- *Have to try and deal calmly and rationally, and try to work with the idea that you are not the problem you just happen to be there that day. Like a Buddhist, let it go though you, although I am not a Buddhist. Sometimes I respond directly. I do not have a lot of patience of people picking on my staff and I defend them vigorously. Some of them I suggest that I cannot help them and they should go elsewhere for their care.*

- *Spend the time to educate them. In some cases fired them.*

- *I try and be tougher.*

- *Try to be professional with them and be firm in my convictions.*

- *They come in knowing what the answer is and they don't want to deviate from that answer no matter what. Predetermined. The ones who really want a diagnosis and they are healthy.*

- *They come and go. It's the same kind of patients. I get along with the difficult patients in general. Have a mixture of personalities.*

Q: How did you handle it?

*Sometimes the patient is asked to leave the practice.

- *Only one time I have contemplated sending someone a letter. Unhappy with me, so go somewhere else, I will help you.*

- *I am very straightforward. I had a patient yell at my staff. I said don't treat my staff like that. He had been kicked out of everyone's office. I didn't kick him out. Most of them straightened out. I only made one go. He was a drug abuser. He broke his contract with me. I don't get mad at them. I feel sorry for them.*

- *There are patients that I can work with. I deal with a lot of patients. The ones where it becomes clear that I can't, I read them the riot act and tell them to go away. That is rare. My threshold is a lot higher.*

* Persisting in finding ways to help is another strategy.

- *I am pleasant but stern.*

- *We tell them that we are here to help them. If it is taking a little longer it is because we are helping someone just like we help them. Once they understand they become loyal.*

- *By spending more time with the parents trying to reconcile their differences.*

Q: How did you feel at the time? Looking back on it?

*Sometimes it's upsetting. Sometimes not so much.

- *I would be happier if I had no difficult patients. Struggling with the balance between the idea that a service provider needs to absorb a certain amount from patients/customers and keep a smile on it with the idea that sometimes you just have to tell people where they are at and you are at and engage in truth telling. A balance. Can't have no fuse but can work on having a longer one. Too long a fuse creates anger and depression.*

- *I felt bad. I was not able to convince them to do the right thing. I was not able to get through to them to do the right thing.*

- *Helpless and ineffective. Sometimes there is a greater good than preventing death and progressive illness. Offering a peaceful passage out of this world. Offering families a way to cope with the loss of a loved one. Those have import which we may not fully appreciate when it feels like defeat in the moment.*

- *When you fire a patient you feel sad. When you educate a patient you feel happy.*

- *Uneasy.*

- *Briefly upset.*

- *Annoyed and yet it is comical.*

- *Accepted in any business or profession. Part of it. As far as people who are demanding.*

- *I try to do my best job. Right or wrong or I can't live with myself if I don't do my best.*

- *It feels great.*

- *I am comfortable with my decisions.*

Q: IN GENERAL, DID PATIENTS GET MORE OR LESS DIFFICULT, OR STAY THE SAME, OVER THE YEARS?

* Some doctors said that patients have "Stayed about the same."

- *About the same. When patients are sick they are sick. As you get busier it feels like it is harder to get around to everyone and give everything 100%. Try to do my best usually my family time gets sacrificed. Some days are crazy. I gotta rush.*

- *Similar pattern, different patients.*

- *People are who they are. They are the same.*

- *Stayed the same. No better or worse. I might have implied on rare occasions that we were not on the same wavelength.*

- *I think that it is the same.*

- *About the same. The environment is more difficult. The patients are very decent.*

- *The same.*

- *Pretty much have stayed the same. There has always been that spectrum of patients you love and hate and in between patients you can work with.*

- *They stay the same. Once they think that you are on their side, they are easy.*

* Some of the doctors find the patients easier because they have become more skilled at the doctor-patient relationship.

- *Less difficult. I don't find them so difficult. Sometimes people feel they don't have enough time with their doctor and I stop them and organize it. People come in shot out of a gun. They only got to spend three minutes with a doctor and so they try to do it in two minutes.*

- *People have stayed the same. It's been easier because I am easier at handling them. I don't get into it like I did when I was younger. When I was less experienced and had a patient with depression I thought that it was my job to talk to them for an hour. It's not my job. My job is to figure out where they are at and where they need to go. Meds, hospital therapist, ER evaluation right now. I used to dread having anxiety and depression. I used to dread it if they were on my schedule. Now it doesn't bother me. Same thing with blood in stool and I am thinking about major GI bleed and I assumed a major bleed and now I think hemorrhoid. When I was inexperienced I went to the worst possible scenario and most of the time it is something simple and not an emergency. That has been a great thing for me. I stopped sweating small stuff and most of the time it is small stuff.*

- *Not more difficult. There are more data to go through. We never had those data but we had more sick patients. We have done more prevention in the past 20 years and it prevents disease. They are less difficult.*

- *With time and experience they get easier.*

- *I do not know if the patients have become more or less difficult but my ability to work with them has improved considerably.*

- *Not much of a change. I feel that I have an easier time connecting with them as I become more confident in my own skills and leave my own insecurities behind and I become more open to the story that they are trying to tell me without trying to peg it down to a specific diagnosis.*

- *Less difficult in seven years. It is not that long. Because we build a bond of trust we can exchange more and patients are willing to run with my ideas. We build a relationship.*

- *Stay the same. People are who they are. Some of them soften when they see that it is not a confrontational relationship.*

- *Definitely easier. You have more experience to fall back on. More tools in my tool kit than I had 30 years ago. I am never never afraid going in to the room and I am never afraid what to do. I will always figure out something to do or some next step not necessarily afraid that I won't know the diagnosis.*

* Patients have become more difficult for several reasons.

- *I have seen my patients for a long time. People are ruder and less respectful than they used to be. My patients have implicit faith, they just do it. No internet, no second opinion. Blue collar people have more respect. And they pay their bills and don't give you a hard time. They don't do insurance fraud. I will look at articles, it helps to explain things to the patient, not to be an autocrat. Have to come to some kind of agreement. This is what I think that this is what you think lets come to some agreement. MD stands for medical doctor – not your mommy or daddy. I say do it or don't do it. You have to have a game plan and be somewhat definitive, we can talk about it or whatever. Sometimes you have to be the mommy or daddy.*

- *Patients are becoming more and more litigious.*

- *If they are difficult, they continue to be difficult unless something really goes wrong and their diagnosis changes.*

- *More difficult. Or more difficult parents have come out and new parents are besieged with so much information. Looking for information online in the wrong places. The very demanding and entitled patients are the hardest. I go to Haiti and work with poor people and then I go to the nursery and people are complaining. Entitled, obnoxious, challenging. Difficult to stay calm with them. I don't like abusive men who tell their wives what to do or who won't let the women have meds because it might hurt the baby if they are breastfeeding.*

- *Some got more difficult. Some trusted me more. Some got sicker.*

- *Patients are getting more difficult as they are receiving incomplete educations from the internet and therefore believe that they have an answer to an unknown questions.*

- *A lot more difficult because there is so much information on the internet. Patients are diagnosing themselves, getting little bits of information from everywhere and other doctors. It's difficult.*

* Sometimes insurance issues make it more difficult, not the patients.

- *More difficult. They have been empowered by the insurance companies and Mr. Obama.*

- *People are the same more or less. But circumstances change so they react. Life, meds, tests are more expensive. They pay more insurance and get less. This builds up frustration, understandably.*

- *The patients are no more difficult. The insurance companies and pharmacies are the problem. The hoops we have to go through to get them what they need. The insurance companies won't allow it even if they need it. Sometimes I can't get an MRI for a patient even if it is what they need. Sometimes I have to settle for one medication when it might be okay when I know that the one that they really need would be better but the insurance company won't approve it.*

Q: Please describe your favorite patient/s. Why?

* Some of the doctor interviewees really connect with certain age groups.

- *I have a lot of favorite patients. I really like my elderly patients. They are really cool. I like my adolescents. They are interesting. I have people that I really like. I see them on my list and I feel good. I have a girl, her mother, her grandmother.*

- *People with a sense of humor even when they do not feel well. I like the older patients. They have a lot to tell you about.*

- *Most of my older patients are my favorite patients. And blue collar. Retired. They are very grateful for the care that I give them. They are nice. I have a few husbands and wives married for 50 plus years and they come in together and it is nice to see the way they treat each other. I may have gotten them better from something serious or I made a diagnosis that helped them live longer or better and they are very grateful. With one woman I picked up an ovarian cancer and she survived for five years and she was very grateful, as was her husband, and that was a rewarding patient for me.*

- *The ones who listen and who I feel really trust me. And appreciate me. Today I saw some. Some of my elderly patients who have reached 100 and I have been to their birthday parties.*

- *I like young adult patients. They are just starting out. It's a nice stage of life. They are generally pretty well and appreciate telling someone they can go to with problems. I like women in my age group. It is very comfortable.*

- *I like dealing with women my age. I think I'm really good at it. I experience the same things. I am not always calm.*

- *So inspiring. The elderly women and men who have the blessing of having their mental faculties. They just need help with the plumbing so that their bodies can keep up with their minds. Age is no impediment.*

- *I don't think I have an anecdote of a favorite patient. Someone who is appreciative is great. Fascinating is who regales you with interesting patient stories and is happy with what I do. I have learned more from people without those qualities who radiate goodness, generosity and contentment regardless of whether they have a dollar in their pocket and are able to communicate it. I am fascinated by the very old patients who are still optimists. I have become a very old optimist groupie.*

* Working together, having been through tough times and coming through it together, doctor and patient, is so important.

• *When they are interested in their problem.*

• *Usually the ones who have had a life-threatening illness and I have saved and I have gotten close to them personally in ways that are almost on the level of a real close family member.*

• *A young guy in his 30s who came to me after a diagnosis of melanoma in the eye. He was just getting worse and his oncologist hadn't told him that he was going to die. So he kept getting chemo. I called his oncologist. So I ended up telling him. I was crying and it was devastating. It was so sad. It was the worst. And basically I was telling him to stop and go on hospice which was a conversation that should have been had with him six months earlier. He died six weeks later. We have patients who die all the time. We are internists and we see them until 90 or 100 and they die. When young people have a diagnosis that should have been detected and they die. Those are the worst. Someone terminally ill or dying before their time.*

*Sometimes appreciation or the relationship itself is the most important factor.

• *The ones with whom I have had a long-term relationship. They have been with me years and years. They are the best. They trust me and they know that I am doing everything to help them that I can. It comes back to that relationship. It's everything.*

• *There are patients that are not always very appreciative of things that are not even important. You may not have done a lot for them but they are appreciative of little things. On the other hand, patients who you have done a lot for and don't hear anything.*

- *I just told you about the one who I took the personal time and thanked me. Two human beings connecting. You cannot kick me around and expect me to give you me good services.*

- *I like most of them. They have a limited life span as a patient. We fix them and they get better.*

- *The ones who like me and they trust me and I look forward to seeing them even years later and don't mind running into them on the street.*

- *They express their gratitude. Give me a gift at Christmas.*

- *The ones who have been through something bad with me, who have done well and changed their lives and are with the program and are interesting and friendly. A lot of them have interests that are interesting to me. For example, cycling. Well traveled and well read. These people are really interesting. Sometime I only find out things through obituaries. I don't have time to get to know them extremely well, but if I have seen them for 10 years, I get to know them.*

- *Second generation who I have known for so long. Not obnoxious or not demanding. Answer their own questions and needed confirmation.*

- *I like patients who are transparent and humble and approachable and don't have a problem with image and tell me what is going on.*

- *The people who live in town my age have kids my age and give me insight about raising kids here and college.*

- *Patients who are willing to engage and want to know stuff. They are hungry for what I have to offer. It brings out the teacher in me.*

- *A handful I really enjoy seeing. They are respectful and they value our relationship. Intelligent but compliant. It's a pleasure dealing with people like that.*

- *Numerous. Not one or two. Just who they are. Just nice people. All different ethnicities and sexual preferences.*

- *It is very hard. I feel like a parent in that I like the vast majority of my patients. I like to help them get better. I don't help everyone so I try to find the next person to help. I love seeing chronic pain patients who have gotten much better because of acupuncture.*

- *All my patients are my favorite patients. I can't really pick just one. I guess my favorite patients are when I provide care to their entire family because I really get to know them. Frequently, I provide care to two or three generations and they are like my family.*

- *Grateful, trusting, and knowledgeable.*

- *The ones who show that they really understand the working relationship that you have with them, and are co-creators of this relationship. They take responsibility for contributing to the relationship and you come up with it together.*

- *They actually care about getting better. They are clear in their complaints and they actually listen.*

- *Two types. People who bring a smile to my face or I feel like we are friends. Soul mates, we just connect. We speak the same language, we speak the same. It's easy to have a conversation. I am not monitoring what comes out of my mouth. It is ok. Like a favorite course. Self gratification like eating a chocolate bar. The other that one is you know that you made an impact on their lives. You know that you are helping them and of course it is nice when they also feel that way.*

- *I like good people. I have known them for years. I really like them. They good work hard and I respect them and they respect me for the fact that I am working hard.*

- *All patients are very unique and it is hard to single out people. Every person is very special in their own regard.*

- *I have so many responsible, respectful patients in my practice. They are nice they understand and they are compliant and listen.*

- *People who let me help them get well and then let me share in their lives.*

Q: IS THERE ANYTHING THAT YOU HAVE NOT BEEN ABLE TO FORGET? ANYONE?

* My interviewees had some powerful stories to tell. One doctor interviewee said, "One amazed me. She was going to have a baby who she knew would not live. It had terminal congenital issues. She carried it to term, delivered it and held it while it died. I see strengths in other people I know I would not have myself." One doctor interviewee answered in a very interesting way, "Why would there be anything I would want to forget?" Many of the answers were remembering patients who had died.

- *When I was a resident. A guy came in with no blood pressure. I thought he was on something. He came into the surgery service. The surgery resident had an idea and tried it. In those days no test to diagnose that he had fluid around the heart. Today you do an echo. No ultrasound yet. Two minutes later the guy went into cardiac arrest and died. I should have stopped and taken him. I wasn't quick or definitive enough. He just walked away. He killed him and I did nothing to stop him. Not quick enough or definitive enough. I try and save people. I have seen people die. We didn't have the knowledge or equipment that we have now. This has bothered me. This is the only time I saw someone killed. He just walked away. "He was going to die anyway." They were lazy. No technology. Other procedures. No CT scan or ultrasound yet. None of us were good at these tests. Do no harm above all. Have to learn and keep the patient in mind and do what is best for them. Never be afraid to call for help. Just help.*

- *There are lots of patients. If you show me a name I will tell you how they died and I feel like if we had done something different and they would still be here. It sticks with you. Others did better than expected for them and survived longer than they were supposed to. I get invitations to wakes and funerals. They accepted me their inner circle.*

- *I remember everything. The ones who passed away. We talk about them and remember them and remember hilarious things that happened. It is a frequent topic of conversation. Our practice is nice. It makes me feel good. I couldn't forget one woman with a complicated disease died as complication of a biopsy procedure.*

- *The vision that repeatedly comes to me when he nurse called and said the patient is no more. His hands are still warm but he was gone. Too many losses.*

- *The cases that were in court. Some of my early AIDS patients. Nothing was known. One patient had lesions around his anus. He presented with urinary retention. When I spoke to the urologist. I told him that I had ordered the AIDS test he praised me. He was a 30-year-old. It was before treatment. Then I had the 50-year-old guy who was sick. He was married with kids and he admitted going to the bath houses in New York. Just had an outer circle friend has been coming to see me over the years. He has hypertension and urology issues. He wanted to stop drinking and wanted to go inpatient. They did blood work. He has hepatitis B. He is just showing symptoms at the same time. In our circle of friends people have said that they wouldn't be surprised if he was bisexual. His wife is also a patient and it is more complicated because he's in the circle of friends. My father said that 50% of all family medicine is psychological. A professor in school used to talk about energy and solar plexuses. Each patient takes a little energy. At the end of the day you get tapped out.*

- *People dying on you. You don't forget them. Many people come to mind when I see their children and the parents have passed on and I spent 20 years taking care of them. So many of them.*

- *Various patients along the way. Staff people along the way. Other doctors. Many people along the road who stand out positive or negative.*

- *Certain patients stand out. I have colleagues who have died who were influential. My son will say this is the reason that he went into medicine. He witnessed an incident in school where a classmate's life was saved.*

- *That patient I just told you about who died the horrible death. The patient who committed suicide.*

- *I remember most people. No one truly memorable.*

- *Yes I have patients who are gone who I don't forget.*

- *There are patients that you never forget. Have really close relationship and then they die. Especially there really sick ones when you are their advocate and then they die.*

- *I don't forget patient stories. I remember everything.*

- *I have vivid memories of my patients. I can push them to the backburner for a while. I can instantly bring them to the forefront if something similar happens. I can see faces. It's not just one patient. What saddens me is to see lives wasted unnecessarily.*

- *Yes. I remember in medical school a young man with epilepsy who fell in Central Park and had a traumatic brain injury. His family donated his heart, lungs, kidneys, pancreas, liver. I was there at the harvest. I will never forget when the anesthesiologist walked away because there was no respiration anymore. All of the organs were harvested. He was gone. I realized how quiet the room was. No heart. No beeps. I looked down and saw the cross his mom had put on him. I went home at 3 am and cried for hours.*

- *The quad patient comes to mind. In her 20's. She lives on her own. Married after the accident. Lots of patients. One amazed me. She was going to have a baby who she knew would not live. It had terminal congenital issues. She carried it to term, delivered it and held it while it died. I see strengths in other people I know I would not have myself. Medicine is chock full of that stuff.*

- *That happens every once in a while. I think of a kid we deliver or a mother. One kid had a bad heart defect. I always wonder if he'll be here in a year. Can't deal with it.*

- *So many good people. My mentors. Still some doctors are my heroes. Role models. I will never forget the help I got. I work in the system where I trained. Some of them are still around. What I do right, I can thank who I emulated. Great doctors and nice people. I also can't forget the long hours and the calls. And some people who have died.*

- *There are always people who make an impression. I don't re-member everyone. I have helped so many people. When you do something a little bit different at 1 in the morning you remember. Or ER five hour operations. People you learn from.*

* Particularly difficult clinical situations are remembered as well.

• *One person died with a headache and the family sued the hospital but I had to testify.*

• *I had a kid who was my patient for six months with a weird presentation, hard to figure out. They were totally non-complaint. The child had cancer. They were not compliant. Fortunately, I had documented everything so I was not sued. I can still see the child. It was examined by three boards. One senior surgeon was supportive, others distanced themselves. They reviewed it themselves and said that no one could have made this diagnosis until months in. I won't forget that I missed a diagnosis that lead to his death even thought there was no way to make it earlier. My chairman and my partners took three steps back. One doctor told the parents that if he, himself, had stayed with them, the child wouldn't have died.*

• *I remember the borderline patients who I dismissed from my practice. No one would take them.*

• *One family filed a law suit that was so vague. They came once. No one could figure out why they sued so the suit was dropped. So it was dropped without prejudice. It was filed two days before the filing deadline.*

• *A lot. I wish I could forget some things. We did research on pot. Now there is too much THC and patients are coming in with panic disorder.*

• *I remember a number of patients. A spectacular failure on my part to fix it or the patients were particularly good.*

- *You never forget the people with bad problems.*

Misc

- *It was now that I am older. Looking back at my 20s when I was so focused and committed and anything was going to stand in my way of being a physician. My parents were so steadfast behind me. Moral support, depressed, overwhelmed. Without them I could not have done it. So much sexism etc. 80s.*

Q: WHAT ROLE DOES MENTAL HEALTH PLAY IN HEALTHCARE?

* According to the American Psychological Association and the American Academy of Family Physicians, well over half of patient visits to primary care physicians are for mental health concerns. Providing mental health care reduces medical costs, and impacts physical health, never mind improving quality of life. A recent study showed that "Childhood stress may raise risk for diabetes, heart disease in adulthood." A Gallup poll revealed significant costs to the workplace in terms of absenteeism and underperformance at work due to mental problems. Combined with the destruction of our mental health and the resulting unavailability of mental health services in this country, this is a serious problem and drain on our healthcare system and economy. I co-authored an article with others in the New Jersey Psychological Association which documents the insurance abuses in denying mental health care. It can be downloaded from my website http://www.dreggyrothbaum.com, under "Writer". Please note that this study only included people who had purchased mental health benefits; they just had trouble accessing them. What about people who have no insurance coverage? What is the point of having mental health parity laws, where mental health care benefits are comparable to with medical healthcare benefits, if the insurance companies deny and refuse to honor existing coverage? The Community Mental Health System and agencies which provide free or low cost mental health services have all but disappeared or have been gutted due to funding shortages.

* No disagreement here for this question, among the interviewees. "A big one." Mental health affects physical health directly as well as via compliance. And another interviewee said, "It's such a huge role. It takes us half of every day." Another one said, "Sometimes we can't do the medical piece because of the mental health piece."

• *Major role. Get depressed. Lose a child or pregnancy. Become overwhelmed. Different life changes. Marriage, divorced , dating scene. A lot. Disappointments that come with that.*

• *I have a lot of people who are depressed. Anti depressants and they won't see a psychiatrist. So I send them to a psychologist so someone will talk to them. I sit and listen. I have known them for 25 years.*

• *Very important. If they have mental health issues anxiety or stress it can cause other health problems. Stress is not good for anyone. How do you un-stress yourself? You have to find ways to do it. Massage, walk away. Find a way to do it.*

• *You can't separate mind and body. When someone has some kind of illness, especially overwhelming or chronic it causes mental health issues. You have to be prepared for it. Part of training and experience. Some people refuse to take their medication and their diseases get worse. Denial. I tried to get her help. She won't go. Commonplace.*

- *A significant effect on health care. Patients who are psychologically unhealthy hurt themselves, abuse their bodies, and increase health care costs in general. Can't separate the mind from the body. It has a major effect and society wants to deny the existence of mental health problems being such a significant part of what occurs of what occurs in this society causing physical ailments. It's so taboo. It's the thing you just don't want to talk about.*

- *A larger one than anyone admits.*

- *Huge. We don't have the resources in the practices to handle it. We as generalists don't have the training to manage the amount of bipolar, ADD, ADHD, OCD, PDD, depression and you can't get the insurance to pay. I had therapy myself and it helps.*

- *A large role. You cannot separate out mental and physical health.*

- *Over all. It's such a huge role. It takes us half of every day. Anxiety and depression, chest pain shortness of breath.*

- *Sometimes we can't do the medical piece because of the mental health piece. It takes a long time and there are multiple layers. Deal with this before that. You can't start at that actual or presenting problem yet. The difference is in how we get information, and then what we can do with it. Is the kid trying to get the attention of the parents or dad is beating mom? Or he is so depressed? Some of our families have never been in this position before. One family has half of their kids with a chronic health condition and the dad lost his job.*

I know what the advice is for the physicians: widen the lens and see people as people even if it takes five more minutes in the beginning. How do you do this with nine minutes per visit? We can only fix it from the medical side. How do you teach medical people about the mental health?

- *Splits within my own abilities. Psychological as much time I would allow them to talk or referred to a child psychologist if I couldn't relieve them of their anxieties.*

- *I find that it plays a major role. Physicians who ignore it will find that compliance deteriorates. If you don't understand your patients' mental health they will not follow up or f ollow your instructions.*

- *Huge role. If they don't feel good they don't take care of themselves. Parts of your body hurt.*

- *Mental health is imbedded in healthcare. A subsidiary but cannot separate it from health.*

- *It should play a larger role. Can't get an appointment with a psychiatrist. I try and make referrals. Insurance won't cover it, you can't find someone to see and there is a stigma.*

- *A big role. They have depression and anxiety. Anything you do here they are happy. Hard to find good therapists and no one is in network.*

- *A huge role. So many things that we deal with are driven by mental health issues. I have a lot of trouble getting patients to go to mental health professionals. Need a psychologist and a psychiatrist.*

- *A big role. Mental health is no different than hear disease or diabetes. It has to be recognized and treated.*

- *I feel like the truly vast majority of patients' complaints are related in some part to their mental health. The day to day stresses, anxieties, depressions all color the self-perception of patients' illness. Since we filter, their symptoms are filtered through the lens of anxiety. We are then affected by their mental health as we filter through our lenses. No easy solutions to most of the stressors of our modern life. If people could decrease their stress, they would. Don't want to use it as an excuse, no cause or cure. I am huge fan of therapy. Cognitive behavioral therapy fits my personality.*

- *Extremely important.*

- *Mental health and the doctor-patient relationship. Patients need to understand better – this is psychology – there is no such thing as a purely physical symptom. Every single physical sensation is associated with emotion and vise versa. It is measureable the immune system. Every time you have a thought your body reacts. Gut feelings, butterflies in the stomach, etc. With a sudden strong emotion water comes out of your eyeballs. It's not imaginary and you have no disease. Mind and body react everywhere, holistically. It's not a vacuum.*

- *If a child or patient has a psychological or neuropsychological problem, I refer to a pediatric psychologist or neuropsychologist. I love talking about theirproblems, but I can't treat them.*

- *Pivotal. Central. Can't put it more bluntly.*

- *A huge role. It decides whether the patient seeks help or gets in the way of getting help and they get in their own way. Huge issue of somatization, which in many ways you cannot uncover from a medical point of view. Many times they go hand in hand.*

- *Not enough. If you have depression it should be treated and maybe not with medicine.*

- *It is totally intertwined with what goes on. I don't even leave it off any more it is another organ system like the heart kidneys and stomach. I would say 40–50 percent of the patient have some mental component to their health. Thirty percent of visits have some emotions involves. Ten percent of the visit is why they are there. Anxiety or whatever. People are more willing to come in and talk about it. It's like erectile dysfunction. First we had a medication and now there is the stigma is off. People who are anxious or depressed don't worry about it. Stigma is removed and we have treatments.*

- *It's very important. I make referrals. I will treat certain disorders myself. Depression. Grief reactions. I know my limits.*

- *That is why people decide to be compliant or not or blame others for their problems. You can get amazing victories when it is improved.*

- *Mental health and mental illness is a topic unto itself. State of mind impacts health. You have to get the patients' perspective. If there is a depressed patient comes in, they may not recognize that it has an effect on another condition. Depression; may not recognize it or they may be in denial that they are having symptoms of depression or may be very resistant to seeing a mental health professional. Try and form an alliance with the patient. It is their choice in the end. The goal is not just to write a prescription, but the medication needs to go alongwith therapy. The healthcare system comes into play, there may be no coverage or there may be limited providers to treat them.*

- *Treating mental illness. Making diagnoses. It has a positive affect – people treating the mental illness.*

* Insurance causes problems with access to mental health care, just as demonstrated in the New Jersey Psychological Association study already mentioned.

• *I have been disappointed in it. Psychiatry. Drugs have limited value. Therapy is of value. But it is an unreimbursable commodity as insurance does not cover it. Some of these problems are intractable. I have had personal experience with someone who had borderline personality.*

• *It's an important part. But the insurance companies who have separated it. The insurance companies make their referrals not me. It is foolish. It has always been segregated and help in a separate light from physical health.*

• *Another area of great need and broken-ness. It is hard to find good care. Reimbursements are low. Licensing and preparation to reach to that point where you are qualified is a very difficult task. So we rely on church, family, counseling.*

Q: DID YOU HAVE ANY TRAUMATIZED PATIENTS? WHAT KINDS OF TRAUMA?

* Overall, yes. Many different kinds of trauma.

• *A lot. Sexual abuse. Domestic violence. Drug abuse.*

• *Head trauma.*

• *By life in general. They had a bad break. Lost jobs. Good people. Everyone is human and we all do something wrong at some point. Scared to go back out and live life. And sometimes their medical issues play a large part of it and their disease is a part of it. It's big adjustment. Sometimes they act out and are angry. Some people do the opposite and regress and decline faster. People who have a good support group at home do better. People who are alone, divorced and had some difficult experiences in life don't handle it well. You add a little extra on them and it tips them over.*

- *Many with physical and emotional. Yesterday one patient whose daughter was really sick and scared her mother to death.*

- *My patients I do not find traumatized by medical experience. They are traumatized by hardships in their lives. Death, divorce, financial ruin, infidelity, estrangement, death of a child. They don't talk about trauma in the medical system. They are open and talk about it. I hear a lot about it because I give the patients a time to talk about it. A lot of doctors don't give them the time and don't explore emotional health and how they feel about themselves.*

- *Yes I had a patient from motor vehicle concussion and anoxic brain injury. But she has done extremely well, some spasticity, very pleasant , smiley. Very bad neuropathy and it is a struggle to fight exhaustion and fatigue. But the smile from her face keeps her and me motivated.*

- *Certainly. Everything from PTSD from the Vietnam War to patients who have not gotten over the death of their children. That I find the worst. I have an 83 year old patient and her son died 20 years ago. The son was grown 40-50 years old. People function. She still is not functioning. Some people you would never even know it. One of my patients was witness to the shooting at a shopping center and got blood on them. Upset but did really well.*

- *What kinds of trauma? I take care of really sick patients. Aids, STDs, rape, cheating husbands giving them HIV. Sometimes this has led to divorce. It's awful.*

- *Kids who have had to be catheterized. Adhesions ripped open by others. I used to see more kids who have been sexually abused but not now.*

- *I am almost sure that a good percentage of my depressed patients are traumatized. A large number of PTSD who did not come from Afghanistan. Just the trials and tribulations of everyday life.*

- *Almost everyone is traumatized. So many people I treat for anxiety and depression. A lot of young people too. And I think that part of the problem is in school we tell our children they are special and everyone gets a trophy. When they come out, no one cares about them.*

- *It created splits within my own abilities. Psychologically, they used as much time I would allow them to talk or I referred to a child psychologist if I couldn't relieve them of their anxieties.*

- *I did a lot. All patients who have been in ICU have PTSD. I have a patient who just came back from Afghanistan. He has panic attacks. He punched his dad at night. You have to go over it and over it. You cannot get tired of hearing it.*

- *Dissociative Identity Disorder. She told me. She came as the personality in charge. I met several of the personalities. Her parents were devil worshippers. She was a victim of cult abuse. I knew to ask for the main personality. She was a teacher.*

- *Losses. Still kind of struggling with grieving.*

- *Sometimes they are traumatized. Many have emotional disorders, psychiatric disorders, troubled family relationships. I am value neutral.*

- *I don't do trauma in the ER. A couple of my patients are war veterans and some cope better than others. Some never recover. I have older patients who are not being physically abused by their kids, but are emotionally abused. Trying to take their house away. Patients ask me to help them fight their families. I feel terrible but here is a limit to what I can do. Surviving a cardiac arrest is a trauma. A lot are depressed and frightened of life. The lucky ones over time will get over it. I try hard to help them get over it.*

- *Lots in the ER.*
- *Accidents. Fire. They are hard. I am trained well. Hemophilia. He had aids and hepatitis C. He never complained.*
- *I am sure that I have emotional trauma. Difficult families, alcoholic parents. They have depression etc., raped at 20 and are now 70-75 and it comes up in conversation not infrequently.*
- *I work in the ER.*
- *Both physically and mentally traumatized.*
- *Sexual and abuse in general.*
- *Sexual abuse. A very high percentage. Women tend to be very repressed. But even these women are more likely to be able to face feeling, but it is harder for them. I may be able to get at it. Sexual abuse, we have to ask about it. Domestic abuse and violence. Patients who internalize abuse issues and it becomes somatic.*
- *Physical trauma. Victims of trauma or accidently subjected themselves to trauma or brain injury. Breaks my heart when I have to take care of a child who accidently overdoses. Or patients who have tried to kill themselves by jumping off a roof or throwing themselves in front of a car or bus. OD on heroin. Pharm party. It's difficult. Devastated and vegetated or mildly cognitively impaired. They all have lasting scars even if they return to baseline physically. Emotional scars.*

- *My male gay HIV patients. My younger patients with severe complications that I have to deal with major life issues. Patients with childhood abuse, spousal abuse. Addiction abuse. The inability of the system to meet their medical needs.*

- *Sexual abuse. Physical abuse to them or their children. 9/11. A lot.*

- *Rape patients. I have more patients where the spouse has cheated. Or have other physical trauma.*

- *Physical, family, emotional, mental. Some of it comes right out. Some it comes out years later. Some of it I find our serendipitously. Some I am taking care of and have never shared it with me.*

- *Hit by cars. In car accidents when they lost their patients. One 12-year-old kid's mother had a seizure and she grabbed the steering wheel and saved their lives. After 9/11 I had a kid who came in with his father. By the time they brought the kid for a recheck the father was dead. He was a fireman. We saw so many of these people. I like firemen and policemen. I like taking care of them. They are so nice. They are salt of the earth.*

- *Every person experiences trauma and some handle it well and some have worse situations but you try to help them as best as you can.*

- *Physically and emotionally abused patients.*

- *Several, more, families who have these complex medical conditions. Very amazing and impressive about how the families have pulled all of their resources to take care of their loved one at home and become so knowledgeable over time. When you see them they have a positive attitude, smile on their face, complying with every aspect of treatment. Surely there must be a lot of stress, but they are so on top of things. These patients energize me. There are a good number of them.*

- *Child abuse. I had 10 over the years. Physical abuse. Mandatory reporting started in 1970. Had a few that were suspicious. Called DYFS. Most of the time the parents were angry. One time the mother called to thank me. "Thank you for getting him out of the house. In a few months I would have killed him."*

Misc

- *A few, not many.*

Q: DID YOU HAVE ANY PATIENTS WITH **B**ORDERLINE **P**ERSONALITY **D**ISORDER**? D**ESCRIBE PLEASE**.**

* Borderline Personality Disorder (BPD), according to the National Institute of Mental Health (NIMH), is a style of feeling and behavior marked by unstable moods, behavior, and relationships. From the point of view of a practicing psychologist, it is often learned from being traumatized. As NIMH further states, most people who have BPD suffer from problems with regulating emotions and thoughts; impulsive and reckless behavior, unstable relationships with other people. People with this diorder also have high rates of co-occurring disorders, such as depression, anxiety disorders, substance abuse, and eating disorders, along with self-harm, suicidal behaviors, and completed suicides.

* The way this may look in everyday life, for example in a doctor's office, is that the person is demanding, super critical, unforgiving, pits people against each other, cannot tolerate disagreement, talks behind peoples' backs, sees most people and situations in absolutes or

"in black and white" or "right and wrong", gets angry quickly and over relatively minor issues, takes unwise risks, is unforgiving and holds grudges, and other such behaviors. Unstable family relationships may increase a person's risk for the disorder. Impulsiveness, poor judgment in lifestyle choices, and other consequences of BPD may lead individuals to risky situations. Adults with borderline personality disorder are considerably more likely to be the victim of violence, including rape and other crimes. This vulnerability also makes these patients a challenge to treat in psychotherapy and they are a challenge for doctors too. It is often quite sad. They need help, but their insecurities and vulnerabilities make it difficult to settle into receiving the help that they need. They are really suffering.

* Most of the doctor interviewees have these patients in their practice. As one doctor interviewee said, "Yup."

• *Maybe. We try to be patient with them. Some end up leaving.*

• *I do, they are horrible. Those and the people who are so narcissistic. They are all in or all out. You are the greatest of the best or you are the worst and not on their side. The psychiatrists have no success with them.*

• *Yes. I haven't faced any personality issues, they are okay with me. But when they call on the phone they are completely different. Our staff is pretty well trained to handle those kinds of patients.*

• *I do. I guess I am not sure exactly the definition but I have patients who are difficult to handle. They are difficult and they can be manipulative like they try to turn around what I say. I seem to have a lot of crazy patients. Birds of feather flock together. Or I try to be nice and so they stay.*

- *I've had them but I tend not to keep them. How much should I try to have this patient like me?*

- *A lot of them. They scream at the staff. And they quit. It is so rude.*

- *Thy tend to show up with abdominal pain. They have been through the whole gamut of work up and they come to me as a last ditch effort.*

- *Yes. One minute they are all over you. You are the best thing since sliced bread. I always warn people if they have been to three other practices you are next.*

- *I know the term. I don't think I understand it. I will say that in medical school, psychiatry was the area where I felt the most powerless. The worst of the worst are in-patient. I didn't know what to say to them. A quarter of my patients see me for depression and anxiety and see me for medication. Some need to be taught stress management and how to cope.*

- *Probably. One guy married and divorced four times. He's a psychopath. He's demanding. I gave him 30 days to find a new doctor.*

- *Yup.*

- *Yes. They are the nasty ones that I get uncomfortable with.*

- *My last one fired me last year. It was ridiculous. Every medicine had to be perfect and she was sensitive to it. They sent a brand name and she attacked me and wrote scorching emails as if I had killed her family. The punishment outweighed the crime. If she put that much into something like this what would happen when I made a real mistake, which I will, because I am human.*

- *I only experience them as difficult personalities. The relationship doesn't go beyond that and I don't deal with it as part of a therapeutic interventions.*

- *One came in for pre-op and then in for a consult. Low IQs with difficulty following directions. Family members who are disruptive. As there is some cognitive decline and they depend even more on the family members. You assume that the family will tell you what is going on but sometimes they don't and it is difficult to figure out.*

- *Probably. I send most of them to psych.*

- *I don't focus on it. If I need help I try to get a psychiatrists involved. We just take care of the problems.Sometimes people come in with a psychological problem looking to fix it with a procedure.*

- *Never formally diagnosed them, I may suspect it. The nice thing is it is a delight to be worshipped. The bad thing is knowing that the worship phase always comes to an end in a fiery explosion of anger, hatred, dismay, and frustration. It is like other things in life, it doesn't last forever.*

- *Yes. We have passive aggressive patients, some bipolar patients. But more often we are dealing with acute or chronic anxiety and depression.*

- *Not that I notice. I had a few bipolar patients.*

- *Not sure. Can't describe it. They are the most difficult to deal with. Patients who are depressed or have a history of abuse. When they develop insight they really move along and make progress. Patients who are feigning insight but they don't have it, and they keep coming back over and over again. You point it out. They say "wow," but they do it over and over again. They are difficult because they also create a lot of barriers. They ask a question and have a preconceived answer and when they don't get it they keep asking over and over and get really frustrated.*

- *Not directly, only as a consultant because someone else taking care of them. I have to be aware when planning.*

- *I don't delve into it.*

- *Yes.*

- *Zero insight into their problems and they always think fibromyalgia. Depressed is more common.*

- *Yes. They never tell you. It's patients who are pushing. One patient is intelligent but she has chronic pain but she also has a drug dependency issue. Constantly on email with us and it's always a narcotic that she wants.*

- *I suppose I do. I don't pay attention. Some kids, they don't want you to touch them. My staff could tell you. I treat them, then they are gone, we are good. Treat and release. I just have to hang onto them long enough to treat them.*

- *Yes. Self-destructive habits and addictions. Poor choices and loss of jobs.*

- *Sure. They can fake it. They comport themselves in a way that you would never know. Hear from the families. But it's not my problem. Psychiatrists and psychologists, we work with them to handle these problems.*

Q: Do you think that the patients understand how hard it is to be a doctor?

* Most of the doctor interviewees answered "no" to
  this question.

• *No, they have no idea. If I have to go to the hospital, I can be pulled out, 24/7.*

• *No.*

• *No. I don't think that they do. Some patients may know how hard it is. A lot of patients think that if there are 40 patients and they don't put their hand on them and give them medication and they are out and the next one is in they think that anyone can do this so they lose faith. Medi-clinics in the pharmacies are dangerous and miss things and treat things inappropriately and are not really the case.*

• *Most, no.*

• *I don't know if they think about it. They take it as a granted. It is hard to get into medical school and have a practice. They think that once you are there, you did it.*

• *No. Absolutely not. The amount of training, the number of hours that you work and all of the stuff that goes on behind the scenes and the stress of holding people's lives in your hands.*

• *NO, No, absolutely not. All they see is that we are rich. The fact that I took 29 years which was quick to get trained and start making money. The cost was at least one half million dollars to become a doctor. The best years of your life, your 20s, are gone. People never see that.*

• *No. they really don't. They used to understand. Had a more glowing respect. This is special and you had to do something special to get where you are.*

- *No.*
- *Nah. It doesn't bother me.*
- *I don't think that they do. I don't think that they realize about being baptized in the blood of human suffering and what it does to you. The sounds of human suffering in hospitals.*
- *No, definitely not. That's why my kids don't want to be doctors. I am a soft person and I cry a lot.*
- *No.*
- *No.*
- *No. they have no idea. You spend nights up thinking about your patients. Patients call. Patients have my cell phone. That's life. I have to leave the movies if I get a call.*
- *No. I do not. The general view is that doctors are rich and all they want is money.*
- *Not easy to be a doctor. Many patients don't understand that. But I have patients who have professions where it is hard or patients have lost their jobs. People face different challenges. Hard to do a lot of things. The challenge also drew me to it.*
- *I do. I think that people do realize how hard it is to train as a physician. I am not sure that they appreciate the sacrifices that we make to be a physician. When someone wants access to you 24/7 they obviously do not realize that you need some private time.*
- *Not at all.*
- *Absolutely not. They think that I have to be brilliant and that I have a lot of money.*
- *No.*

- *No. The reason why is that I am amazed by the reimbursement received by certain sports players. Physician reimbursement in some cases can be as low as 1/1000 of what they make. People will pay thousands of dollars to see a Super Bowl and then refuse to pay a $25 co-pay. Society's choices for heroes nowadays is very confusing to me. Why are we paying millions for dollars to play a game? People are starving. How do you legitimize it? Look at some of the models. They give some money to a children's foundation. Whoopee. I can't believe that the general public doesn't see it.*

* Some of the patients understand. Sometimes that makes a difference in the way that they behave and sometimes it doesn't make a difference.

- *Yes. But they do not understand how we get paid or the administrative BS we have to deal with. They understand the amount of time we spend getting trained. Physicians are still held in high esteem and trusted. A friend of mine, 70. He has a lot of care. He could go anywhere. But he said he said he trusts my judgment. Gives me positive rewards, especially as a family doctor. A patient with MS wants me to do the quarterbacking and help make the decisions. I have a patient in a clinical trial for cancer and the patient and her husband come to me to help with difficult decisions. The trust is overwhelming sometimes.*

- *Some of them do. Not all of them appreciate it.*

- *Some patients do because they see what you are doing and what time you come to work. They do not understand the business aspect of it. When they get the insurance they see what they were charged but not what it costs. Doctors do not make a lot of money anymore.*

- *Some do. Every once in a while I will run into a patient that is so kind and is so in relation to this and often it will come at the point where I walk in the room and say that I am sorry for being a bit late. And the response will be don't apologize to me you have such a tough job. But my response is that I am there for them. That's the exception by and large they have no idea and don't care how hard it is. Everyone is egocentrically going through life.*

- *Some have insight. But honestly, they don't care. We are a service and they expect a certain level of service and it has nothing to do with how hard you are working. Or they will move on. Unless no one else will give the service, which no one may do one day.*

- *Some of them but not most of them. The people who are less educated don't realize it. If you have not had that responsibility you don't realize what it's like. I gave up my 20s and 30s. When you pay me now you are paying me for all the years that I lived below minimum wage so I have the expertise now to take of care of you.*

- *I think they do and they think it is harder than I think it is. I can refer to someone else and get myself off the hook and it's not too hard anyway.*

- *A lot of them do. I have developed a really nice practice. I like to think that my patients respect what I do for them.*

- *Most of them. Not the borderlines.*

- *Yes and no. Some of them express sympathy and concern for I am working hard. They do not know it directly. Many of them may have worked harder than I do. They may look at me as a fellow traveler. I don't know.*

- *Yes, but so what? If you don't feel well and you are sick you are demanding, you want it now. I get it but it doesn't make it easier.*

- *Some of them do. Not all of them. A lot of my patients see me in the ER and they do.*

- *Our patients are very mindful of the burden that doctors have. My patients have been supportive and helpful. We forget who the real heroes in the system are and I think that it is the patients. They have to deal with their illnesses and the financial strain. They need access to specialized care. They are juggling sickness, work, family.*

- *A minority do. Better than the general public. They see you and what is going on in health care.*

- *Some do. Some think that it is simple and financially rewarding.*

- *No. I love being a doctor. My son is a resident. His interest on his debt is $1000.00/month. But we always need doctors. It has to be saved.*

* Three doctors look at it differently.
- *It is not hard to be a doctor. It is hard running and office, paperwork, fees. I am not anxious about being a doctor or about surgery. I get excited when looking forward to surgery. Patients say it to me all the time.*

- *Most doctors do not understand how hard it is to be a patient. Doctors are well compensated for the labor we provide and I expect no sympathy from my patients. I can quit anytime and do something else. Conversely most patients do not get the choice of being a patient.*

- *It's not hard. I have a nice life. I go on vacation. People like me. They give me presents. I work for myself. My son works for an internet company. Has a quota. When you go to anyone you expect people to be competent and do what they can do. In any profession and that is what the public should expect from me. The same thing with my plumber, or handy man.*

Misc
• *I don't know.*

Q: DOES THE GENERAL PUBLIC?

* The public doesn't understand most of the time either. "The public looks at us money grubbing pigs."

• *No, absolutely not. The public looks at us money grubbing pigs. In some cases they are right. Most of the people I know work hard. People don't wake up and say, "who can I kill today or rip off?" I read the Times and magazines and there are people who do that. I only deal with people who do right. Not because insurance is a piggy bank. I am affiliated with a university. There is scrutiny. They will throw you out. The nurses know what is going on. In the New York Times there are always stories. There is the potential there. If that is what you want to do, you can get away with it. No one is looking for quality. I do not associate with that.*

• *No. I don't think that they do. Some patients may know how hard it is. A lot of patients think that if there are 40 patients and they don't put their hand on them and give them medication and they are out and the next one is in they think that anyone can do this so they lose faith. Medi-clinics in the pharmacies are dangerous and miss things and treat things inappropriately and are not really the case.*

• *I don't think so.*

• *There is something that has changed a bit in becoming a doctor that I didn't have to deal with. Incredible student loans. It is incredible impact. It is a deterrent. You could go to Wall Street or be an attorney. You can't pay them back. It impacts who decided to be a doctor.*

- *Absolutely not. The media is raining down on doctors. Wherever something doesn't go right with health care it is the doctors fault.*

- *No. Most people who don't have a family member who is a doctor I think that you have no idea. Even friends of doctors have no idea how hard it is. Family sees the stressed out decompression phase of the day. I am not much of a drinker but there were times when I would pour a little sip of Jack Daniels. If I have 3-4 drinks in a week it's a lot.*

- *No.*

- *To a certain degree. But they do not understand what is being sacrificed. You have to decide early in life to give up pleasures that other people have for example in college, social activities and sports. Life was around pre-med, science and good grades, people who just graduate and get married, have families and we had to delay life for many years until you finish. You have to understand that this was part of life that you would sacrifice years. Thirteen years for me.*

- *No. They think that doctors should make about $70K per year. If you select them out, you may be disappointed.*

- *No. They do not understand what we face. The lack of reimbursement and the complicated system of dealing with the insurance companies, arguing, trying to get things for them, and you have to fight for your patient and they do not understand how much you are working and how you are fighting for them. With Electronic Medical Records, there is no eye contact. You are typing the whole time. Conversation with no eye contact with you will miss 50% of the story.*

The perception on tv has skewed things. People who are flawed like House. They are brilliant but break the rules. We need Marcus Welby back, I watch the reruns sometimes to remember why I became a doctor.

- *I am sure that they don't know. Why should they? I do not know about plumbers and electricians. I am grateful. I am sure they come across clients that as crazily demanding. I do think that they think that we are all wealthy, especially when they don't have any money.*

- *Absolutely not.*

- *No.*

- *Not in the same way we used to. Still garners respect to be a doctor, but we don't walk on water. Sometimes I think patients would be better off if they still thought that we were the father figures. They need that.*

- *They don't think about it unless they are dealing with a doctor or a feeling. We are the emblem for a failed system. For example, if a patient does not have a referral, you get mad at me, but it is their fault, not mine. There are hundreds of companies and we have no idea if they need a referral. The primary care doctors won't give a referral on the spot. The doctor and the staff get the brunt of it. Calling the Horizon computer does not give you satisfaction, but yelling at the receptionist will give you satisfaction. They still think that the hospital and doctors split the $100,000 bill 50/50. We are not keeping those fees that they think that they are paying insurance cuts it by 80.*

- *Definitely not.*

- *No.*

- *I don't know. I think it's all over the place. Some are culturally driven. I do think it's my impression that the mistrust of doctors and the mistrust of western medicine in general and pharmaceuticals is significantly on the rise. People feel somewhat wanting to be more informed and they act based on being more informed. A doctor's advice used to be trusted, but now they ask Dr. Google and get misinformation and modify recommendations. A tremendous well of information.*

- *Absolutely not.*

- *They see medicine as a prestigious career that is well remunerated and at the height of expectations for their child. They don't understand that you lose your early 20s and 30s, and for women, the opportunity to have children in a rational manner.*

- *No.*

- *It is becoming that we are glorified technicians and not educated practitioners.*

- *Yes, but they are misinformed, mostly by politicians. The representation of the true healthcare needs have been distorted and misguided by insurance, big corporations. They can lose track of the daily struggles of the doctor and the patient.*

- *I don't think so. The complexities are being able to provide the correct care. And the demands on my time. Paperwork. I could be here lots of hours more doing paperwork.*

- *No. I don't think so. I think that the general public and people in general expect a lot: 3 things of doctors: affability, ability, and availability. When not at their beck and call and almost instantly available it's hard to get patients to understand. The whole time I was practicing, there was a tremendous lot patients who never paid their bills.*

* Some of the public does understand.

• *I think they do and they think it is harder than I think it is.*

• *In the rest of the country doctors make more money than their patients. In general the public still thinks that doctors make a lot of money.*

• *They have more knowledge of it now as time has gone on. So much information is available. Both non-fiction and fiction.*

Misc

• *No idea.*

• *I don't know.*

Q: PLEASE EXPLAIN TO ME THE COMPLEXITY OF BEING A DOCTOR. WHY IS THIS SO HARD FOR PATIENTS AND THE GENERAL PUBLIC TO UNDERSTAND?

* Time, and hard work, which is impacted by insurance company problems. "We are used as pawns in a system. No one cares about the doctors."

• *Time management. We have to spend less time with patients now.*

• *They do not understand the mindset of a doctor and the amount of toil and labor both physically mentally and financially that it takes. They do not understand that we have no control as a profession, that others rule us. We are used as pawns in a system. No one cares about the doctors.*

• *It's 24/7. I need a break. Sometimes I don't want to talk about it when I am out and someone walks up to me.*

• *Most people feel that they are entitled to free health care. But they don't understand that the education and the training to become a doctor and the support necessary to run a hospital or that an office costs a lot of money. There is no way we can do this for free. We want equality for everyone, or so we say, but I could bet if there was a free hospital in New Jersey where people who could go for free care. The people who think that they are entitled to the best care would still run to the specialist and pay. We want equality but we really don't. We want a two-tiered system. If no money, not same treatment. The socialist system. Even if you can pay for it you still can't get it. Canada and Mexico come here, they don't like socialist medicine. We provide an enormous amount of free care to illegal aliens. In the setting of a real emergency no doctor would say no. You take care of the patient because you care.*

- *A lot of doctors are no different than plumbers. They do their job and then they are done. Some really care what they do. Not simple, a lot of answers.*

- *The increasing amount of medical knowledge and technology going up constantly and the complexity of the health care system increasing dramatically. Patient knowledge increases dramatically. Good. The amount of time that you have to see a patient face to face is being squeezed by the system, the need to see more patients, the need to do more paperwork and now by the Electronic Medical Records, which is not making things more efficient. It's the opposite so far. Maybe it will change over time. Look at my career in almost 20 years, people who would not have survived are surviving and many times doing well due to the advances in healthcare but it is more challenging to stay on top of things to take care of them. More complex chronically ill patients are being managed at home and require more coordination of care by the doctors and the families.*

- *Is to have the knowledge base which is expanding dramatically. The pressures that come from regulations and different agencies. I am allowed to have a failure rate of 0%.*

*In any other industry you are allowed a failure rate of 0-2%
as the industry norm. I am not allowed that luxury. They
have not done it. It looks easy but a lot goes into it. Like me
when I see a pilot. It looks easy to fly, but a lot goes into it.
Same for medicine.*

• *So many things: the changes in medicine and things to
know medically. And the business part of running a practice.
I like to do things if I can myself. I enjoy it, like computers,
but with insurance and regulatory issues it's becoming
overwhelming. Audits. It's annoying. I am not compensated
for it.*

• *Because most people aren't committed at such a young age
at everything. My kids aren't either. I was so focused in
high school. Women are putting it off, having kids. You
have to be a physician early on. You have to focus early on
or you are already way behind the eight ball. The dedication
and the commitment. The kids in their 20s, they are partying
at night. The people in medical school can't do that. We had
tests. We were sitting in the library or on call. Studying
and studying.*

• *The other part of it is that I didn't even get into following
the rules of the insurance companies. They put pressure
on you. They don't want to approve tests. The insurance
companies subcontract out to other companies who are there
to preauthorize or approve the tests that you order. So it is
almost based on some clinical guidelines of a paper that has
been written. They can always refer back to that. But it is
not always, sometimes it is not correct and they cover do it
just to say no to a test. An example that I can give is that I
had a patient who had an abnormal EKG and I wanted a
nuclear stress test to rule out heart blockage. The patient had*

elevated sugar, high cholesterol and high blood pressure. According the other guidelines of the gatekeeper, if the patient was diabetic it would have been approved. This person was 118 and 120 is diabetes. So I get on the phone with the medical director. In this instance the guy said to me if this guy was fasting and had a donut, that would make the sugar go high. Money savings attempt for the insurance company. This frustrates me beyond all belief. It was a busy day, trying to stay on time. They are watching your utilization. How much money you cost them. Are your patients going to the hospital a lot or getting a lot of expensive radiologist tests? Are you prescribing expensive medication? And while a lot of this is good – I do support older generic medications, they are tried and true, as well as not ordering unnecessary tests – the problem is that there are times when you need tests and the medication that you need does not come generic. So I am spending my day trying to keep the insurance company happy and trying to take care of my patients and keeping them happy. These things do not always work. Sometimes taking good care of the patient does not make the patient happy. They do not want to get a test. That interaction of trying to be a good doctor, while trying to make the patient go along with it and be happy with the plan, while keeping the insurance company happy is the greatest stress. That is it in a nutshell. I could have a great medicine that would be great for the patient, but it is expensive, so the patient doesn't like it and the insurance company doesn't like it. So the patient is asking for an inexpensive medicine and the patient and the insurance company are happy but do not feel like I am doing a good job. My day is a series of compromises.

- *I went to med school after college. Started practicing 13 years after I finished med school. Unless you have the passion for it you cannot be a doctor. Half of your younger years are going into books, calls, and no sleep.*

* "The complexities are being able to provide the correct care," said one interviewee.

• *I don't think that you can understand unless you do it. Everyone expects you to just be for them, people are begging me for a house call.*

• *The 24/7 responsibility and the potential magnitude of problems.*

• *Wearing several hats at the same time. Show compassion but have to know where to draw the line with recommendations.*

• *Until you are immersed in that life you can't really understand. That is your life. People go to work 9-5. Their work doesn't typically impact someone's life. You don't have those nightmares of did this patient do this or that. It's in your brain all the time. It's hard to understand us or sympathize with us. They think that we get compensated for it.*

• *We have so many tests we can't order. The public thinks that we know more or can do more than we can. Ultrasounds don't mean it's a perfect baby. All of the tests and technology moves so fast that we don't know what we see.*

• *The complexity is what I stated in the beginning. It is paramount. You cannot know everything about everything. You have to know what you don't know. You have to decide who needs care and who doesn't. And you have to know where to go. The computer and fax machines and copy machines.*

• *We have the pressure to see more patients. It is all about them, they have the problem and our job is to help them. Two hundred patients a day come through our office. We do a good job in our group. We do stress tests etc. We keep* *hopping but we are efficient. We have an excellent administrator. We provide the Marcus Welby kind of experience to them on an individual basis. Every day I am making decisions. I am not in the OR but I am making decisions about tests and medication. I was also fortunate my parents paid for two years of medical school and I did a fellowship. They paid for college. I came out of medical school with no debt; most people have $200,000. The public does not understand that. And you are not making any kind of significant money until around age 30. Until you have a job. They think that we are rich. The thing about medicine, I am not complaining. I am comfortable, but I am not making like Wall Street guys. I didn't want that. Certainly not in primary care. Mental health is one broken piece. In primary care it's all about relationships. I am hopeful I am making the diagnosis and following up. Those who appreciate how hard it is to do what I do are my better patients.*

- *It is a gradual inculcation into culture. It stared in my first year in medical culture. I did not understand how crazy the culture is until I started working in a hospital. I didn't understand until years of sleep deprivation, people with difficult life experiences, people with trauma. It is a traumatic experience. This training process is rather closed and takes a long time and changes a person 8-12 years before you start to practice.*

- *Underneath it all you are dealing with issues that could affect the patients' outcome of life while simultaneously trying to fix boo-boos and convince people they don't have cancer. You are mother, healer, teacher all in 15 minutes.*

- *The complexities are being able to provide the correct care and the demands on my time. Paperwork. I could be here lots of hours more doing paperwork.*

- *It is hours. To do it right you have to keep learning and keep looking things up. I don't think that the public understands. Sometime I see something I haven't seen before at midnight in the ER. I have an "app" for that.*

- *When you have been a physician for 30 years – I am still training and reading journals.*

- *Integrating the science with the business with the humanism. It is a touchy one. But that is what makes it exciting and rewarding.*

Misc
- *It depends on world view. I used to be a socialist. Anti-free market. Once I started having a business I could see it more clearly. But now I see the country on the fence leaning towards equality versus freedom. Either you make everyone equal and impose it or have freedom. Milton Freeman. There are a lot of crooks; crooks who produce and crooks who destroy. The planters who sweat to plant and the tree shakers.*

- *I think they do understand.*

- *They don't get it. They listen to the media.*

- *There is not a lot of complexity. You go through education and get trained. People have an understanding that it is complicated. I think that they understand that it is complex. But people think you are there and know what you are doing once you go through the process and you are as good as you are going to be. Not true. You get better and better as you do it.*

- *So many of your questions are about how hard it is. I didn't think it was that hard.*

CHAPTER 4

BEING A DOCTOR NOW

Q: Is being a doctor different now than it was when you started?

- *Yes, improvements in clinical medicine. Science advances and we have well trained researchers doing incredible work. It is in the media all the time!*

- *100%. Patients are the same. Treatment and technology has improved. Don't see some of the bad stuff, not bad prostate cancer and colonoscopies. Mammograms. Blood pressure and cholesterol, so many medicines. Lots of good years with cardiac conditions. Diabetes. Treatments are so improved. Losing toes, legs. Vascular disease. Public is more aware of health and health conditions. People are more educated. Internet has helped. I would rather deal with patients actively involved in their health. Some people go overboard. Most people are good.*

- *Yes. Diseases not even known before. Electronic records. What is kind of nice is the patient centered home. It's more interesting and it is a care team with coordinator. The nurses and physician assistants. It's invigorating. I am the captain of the team. The work flow and day to day description is different. It is rejuvenating. It will get me through the rest of my career.*

- *Now it's a lot of talking to patients and communication. In training it was more about increasing knowledge and skills.*

* Many business and insurance changes are for the worse. As one interviewee said, "Gradually as the insurance companies took over they squeezed the doctors. Then came managed care and they managed the doctor. And the doctors were seduced into them. Now we are being seduced into being employees. Now you can no longer advocate for patients or you lose your job."

- *It's different. We covered it. It was only 10 years ago. I was part of a group for a little while. I didn't feel like there was as much. Maybe I was innocent and naïve. Every patient that comes in you didn't think that it could end badly. I was always optimistic. Now I have seen all kinds of people get information first on the first visit (history) and the second visit do something that you would have done on the first visit with less experience. Now I am a little bit more careful and paranoid, hard to live with the fear. I see lawyer l etters. I have seen my friends and good doctors get sued for things that I think that they did correctly.*

- *Yes. For the same reasons. Too many intrusions from insurance and government. Remuneration has not kept up with the times. There was more fat in the practice early on when people had indemnity insurances. Could see more patients with more time. Now, I never changed, but nowadays, I am done with paying for school. I am more interested in enjoying my work. I am not on that merry go round.*

- *All the paperwork and the computerization and it really takes you away from really being with the patient and being with them and examining them closely. Everything is a CT scan and putting things into the computer. If you just spent the time with the patient and listened, you would have 99% of the diagnoses. The computerization and the multiple testing has added but has taken away so much. It's clean and you can read it — it's not scribbled. No question. There is a loss. I used to call every patient with every lab. No there is no time to do that so I have to give it to someone else who has limited clinical experience and wait until the next time that I see them, unless it's really serious.*

- *I have only been out 10 years. It has changed a lot in the last 20 years. It is more business than patient care. It is harder to be out of network. People are already paying so much for insurance.*

- *It's a totally different profession. When a doctor started practicing in the 60s, most were primary care physicians. Why take the time to go into a specialty. The doctor graduates from medical school in the 1960s, most people opened their own practice. No such thing as student debt. Malpractice premium was $100 per year. My office cost me for the medical equipment and the renovation $10,000. Today a doctor graduates with an average debt of $250,000. To open an office is a minimum of $100,000. It's between $15,000 and $100,000 for malpractice. Even if licensing can be rushed it takes three to six months to get credentials by Medicare and the insurance companies. How can you possibly survive with no income and the expenses? 99% will not open their own offices. You will have an income and a patient load day one. Will not have to create new rules and regulations, just see if the office is violating the rules. No such thing as walking in and creating your own private practice. Different mentality. We learned by trial and error, maybe it's better or maybe it's worse. Now the mentality is that you are signing onto a job. HMO, Practice, hospital, etc. I tell them not to let the money be their driving force. Every single doctor gets a job. It's 9-to-5.*

- *Yes. Very different. A lot more regulations in the hospital. More laparoscopic surgery, which is good. Reimbursements. More expenses, electronic medical records, malpractice expenses.*

- *I think yes it is different because there is less respect for doctors than 25 years ago. More administrative paperwork. You are working harder to make less money. Society in general has a litigious nature. Everybody thinks that if something goes wrong sue the doctor.*

- *Yes. All the healthcare changes. My practice has changed from the hospital to office and sub-acute. There is less autonomy at the hospitals.*

- *I still enjoy getting up and going to work but they are trying to make it harder. Yes there is more insurance company control and government control and the computer has changed a lot. Doctors are the smartest dumb people around. We give it away, we let someone else control it. They will stab you in the back. Not thinking of the long term.*

- *No question. The big why is the involvement of insurance companies, both the paperwork and the limitations and they are saying the fee, getting their percentage of it.*

- *Oh yes. I find myself being ignored more than ever by government. A lot of professions think that they just need a license and they can do it. Thirty years of experience. Twenty three years of training. Twelve years of residency. I can do the same thing. Doctors are relinquishing. They were given an incredible gift by our forefathers. When insurance came many of them became seduced by the payments. Driving big cars, belonging to country clubs. You could make a good living. Gradually as the insurance companies took over they squeezed the doctors. Then came managed care and they managed the doctor. And the doctors were seduced into them.*

Now we are being seduced into being employees. Now you can no longer advocate for patients or you lose your job. The hospitals can bill more. We cannot compete with the hospitals. Once I become a hospital employee, if the hospital says no respirator or a morphine drip, you cannot say no. You lose your autonomy, so you lose your profession.

- *It's not that different. I didn't start in the heyday of medicine when I could have a big house and a full time housekeeper and not worry about money.*

- *A little. I was just on the cusp of managed care. There is much more cost containment. The biggest issue is the prior authorizations of tests and medicines. It is so much time that we spend fighting with insurance companies for testing, diagnostics, and therapeutics.*

- *Yes. It is much more regulated than it used to be. The economics have become much more challenging. Issues of limits that we have to deal with or were less of a concern or did not exist 25 years ago. We have to see more patients in the same time. A physical organizational challenge.*

- *I don't think so. I have not been in practice for that long for it to seem different. The fear of what is going to happen. So fearful about the cuts that have happened and are coming. We are considering selling the practice.*

- *Vastly different. The three or four big things: The computer. In a lot of ways it is a huge negative. It is more positive for the overseers. Right now it is gigantic time waster. Letters with filler etc and is not for better medicine. Before there were typed. Now this system does not talk with other systems. Mistakes can be perpetuated easily. It has cut down on face to face time with patients. The eye contact goes. I print it all out onto a paper cart. But most practices have replaced paper with a computer screen. The business aspect is getting harder and harder. So far it has not altered our practice but you never know. People are more stressed out, patients and doctors. New people in the field want hours and salary and to be done with it. That is the expectation. It may not be wrong. How can you tell what you are like at 35 versus 55 and is that the reason it seems different. When I trained we did more on the job training and now fellowships are longer. They have a lot more to learn.*

- *I started in 1966, which is when Medicare and Medicaid started. In simpler times doctors worked it out with the patients. Shifting paradigms. You used to have total care. I took care of you in the office. In the hospital, it's the hospitalist and then the ICU. Fragmentation of care and trying to wire it all together. There is the EMR now to try and coordinate it. The fragmentation issue is huge. I tend to function as the bridge.*

- *It is so different. I stay up every night until one at night on the computer. I am not good at it. I cannot do my charts in front of patients. Computer stuff.*

- *Very much, regulatory insurance and regulatory issues.*

- *Yes. One of my pet complaints is the number of demands on me and my time that have nothing to do with medicine. Insurance and regulations. Less time to do more. That changes practice. Paperwork has to be filled out in a certain way and that is not what I would do.*

- *It is different than when I first started . The whole EMR thing. There're are a lot more women in practice. more in primary care. A lot of female surgeons, OBGYNs. Certain specialties are more male dominated: urology, ENT. In medical schools more than half the students are women. The reimbursements form insurance companies are lower.*

When I came into medicine it was past the days when people were getting rich. There is a lot more information available so that is positive.

- *Not much. A little more of this cost containment things going on now. I started in the era of the HMO. The doctors that were 10 years older than me saw the biggest difference in medicine.*

- *Yes.*

- *Absolutely.*

- *Yes.*

- *Yes.*

- *More of my time is administrative. Not spent with patients.*

- *It's overregulated, over bureaucratic and it is totally screwed up. The public doesn't know they are getting screwed. It's breaking down.*

- *No. Being a doctor is not different. Running a medical practice is totally different.*

- *For sure. Why? Initially I could practice medicine more freely and with better remuneration. I need to live.*

- *So many ways. The doctor-patient relationship is not the doctor in the middle of the insurance company and the patient. Liability and malpractice meant that a really terrible doctor did terrible things and should get nailed. Now medical liability concerns inform every conversation with every patient and every note and you have to constantly think about covering your ass. And it affects the way you practice. If there is a possibility you may feel uncomfortable with not ordering it, i.e., may get a CT scan for a little stomach ache in case it is pancreatic cancer and you might get sued later. It drives up the costs. Not because you are greedy, but you are just covering yourself.*

- *More paperwork. More documentation. More insurance restrictions. Many of these mandates and regulations have been handed to us by the national and state government. These changes have changed the way we practice. We have to be cognizant of the tests we recommend, the procedures that we do. As a physician who cares I am always thinking of how this will affect the family financially. How much will this increase their stress?*

- *I was seeing up to 70 patients per day. It gave me very little time to actually know who the patient was. It was the norm. Then I dropped insurance and changed my style. I do not know how to take care of people without knowing them. Take care of patients in many different ways. This is not the road we are headed down. We are headed down the other road.*

- *Absolutely.*

- *In the beginning, there was just one person in the office. No fax machine. I just had a beeper. I would have to find a phone and pull off the highway. I could never have been this productive back them. I have so much more paperwork. A hospital system is buying my practice. It's too much. All the paperwork. If I read all of the paperwork I wouldn't see patients.*

- *Yes. More team based care. Less doctor-centric. More patient driven. Patients are more responsible for care. More access to information by us and patients. More administrative burden and more regulations. Some of it is good, some is bad.*

- *The technology is different.*

- *Very different. We had fewer patients, the financial part of running a business was okay. Now you have to work hard just to stay afloat. That takes away from interacting meaningfully with other doctors and students. It's very impersonal and very rushed. The ownership has been surrendered to corporations and HMOs where they dictate who their doctor should be, what they should do. A huge intrusions and reduces choices.*

- *It's more demanding. The public expectations. Didn't have to know as much about drugs and genetics. Some medicine is beyond my grasp – biochemical and genomic. The new physicians are not the same. They have a mentality of going to work. And they don't dress up. Same in many ways in biochemistry and pharmacology. They do know more than me. But it doesn't make them better doctors.*

- *It is very different. Paternalistic view of doctors. When I first started people looked on doctors that way and doctors liked it. Answered questions like what would you do? Etc. Now the patient is a "partner" and it is difficult. Medical decisions are difficult.*

Misc.
- *Yes. I am calmer 30 years later. I have seen it before.*

- *Yes. Absolutely. Some things are better. Being a woman is not as weird.*

- *I think it would still be a serious choice. When I made a decision it was somewhat of an emotional decision based on dissatisfaction with things. In a different situation or environment. I might have opted for a different career. But I am not dissatisfied.*

- *It's different but I am different. It's hard to tell what is me and what is the world. When I first started I was newlywed with no kids, so my needs have changed.*

Q: If so, why?

* Business and insurance issues continue to be mentioned. Also, malpractice. As one interviewee said, "Fear of malpractice has changed everything. When I started in 1954 it never occurred to us that we would be sued. We never thought about it or that we would have to protect ourselves by doing an extraordinary number of tests or consultations."

• *Where do I begin? It is different because when I started, patients came to the office, they paid for the office visit. We provided a form to submit to their insurance company. I had no billing costs to speak of and I could focus exclusively on providing care of my patients. Today I have a billing department and an administrative staff to handle our practice. There are more of them than the doctors. Our reimbursement has remained at best flat and more likely decreased over the last 15 years. Costs go up. Fees go down.*

• *Not so much regulations and red tape. Medicine seemed very straightforward. It was just you and the patient without having to deal with all of the other insurance factors that come into the doctor patient relationship, administration, insurance, bureaucracies. The ability to practice without someone looking down your throat. Now you need approval to practice. You are told by others with no experience with medicine how to practice and how to treat. You cannot sometimes give the best treatment to a patient because of bureaucrats who want to tell you to give second best or last best treatments.*

• *I think that the fundamental way I relate to patients and the relationship is the same, or at least we try to keep it the same. Sacred ground. But the functional way that practices work has changed.*

- *Fear of malpractice has changed everything. When I started in 1954 it never occurred to us that we would be sued. We never thought about it or that we would have to protect ourselves by doing an extraordinary number of tests or consultations.*

- *Less engaged with our patients from a hands on approach and more engaged with technology. EMR – they do nothing to improve the health of patients. I can't just flip through a chart and see what I need to see.*

Q: IF SO, HOW?

- *More technology.*
- *It's a violation and makes no points.*

Q: IF SO, WHEN?

- *Probably after 30-35 years ago. The insurance was originally only for hospital care then it became for office visits. Paperwork and money. Trivia – patients knew they didn't have to pay.*

- *A continuous process since I completed my training in 2006.*

Q; HAS PRACTICE CHANGED?

* For example, patient visits are now very short, as a result of the restrictions imposed by insurance companies. One study, by the American Academy of Family Physicians, revealed that it is a maximum of 20 minutes, with most appointments being shorter, yet our doctors are still responsible for providing competent care in that time.

*Again, because of business and insurance issues.

• *I have known nothing but change. First it was fee for service. Then HMOs. In that lawsuit a patient said that I didn't send her for an x-ray because I wanted to make more money from the insurance company.*

• *So many people overseeing you. People don't respect us. What if every single decision has to be justified to a pre-law student with one political science course — to my sister-in-law — by a judge? I spend my day talking to idiots with a book of algorithms. If you say the wrong word they deny the treatment. One guy — insurance on blood pressure meds for 15 years. The insurance company wants to try something else. I had 20 years of medication history. Why switch it now and reinvent the wheel? What if his meds don't work and he has a stroke? Do they want to pay for that? I get paid every day at the hospital but not at the nursing home. Penny wise and pound foolish. So have a stroke and go to rehab. Name brand.*

• *I worked at a clinic first then I came to private practice. All the paperwork is getting worse and worse.*

• *In that what I was seeking early in practice was a very individualized doctor patient relationship in and individual or small group practice. Unfortunately government reimbursement has pushed individual practice out of business and forced us to join large hospital-based practices. Some good things. I have a particular interest in teaching, and working closely with other specialists which you can only do in a hospital setting. Where it has suffered is there is less of an intimate feel of one-to-one relationship with patients. The privacy factor has gone away.*

- *A lot of requirements, government compliance requirements, that deal more with the procedure compliance documentation, clicking the right button. Documenting steps of what you do rather than focus on what is good for the patient and doing it. I spend a lot of my day documentation. It is important but has become onerous.*

- *In my era it has always been having to ask the insurance companies for permission. It may be better because we are now pretending that we matter. It is harder for the specialists.*

- *For the worse. It is more demanding. I enjoy medicine. I probably would but not a primary care doctor. I spent 30 years building up my practice and now I have to turn it over to someone else to run and own.*

- *Practice has not changed. Management has changed.*

- *My practice has changed in that I am looking at doing more other ways other parts of medicine to bring in income. I am looking to branch out into some more administrative work, but it's tricky. I went into internal medicine because I felt like it would give me a lot of variety and I would learn something new every day and not become mundane and not be bored. I like learning and learning new things. High BP diabetes etc but if I get stuck I can talk to a specialist. My days are broken up with different stuff. Not seeing the same thing over and over.*

* Some clinical issues have seen improvement.
- *Yes. Training of docs has changed – beginning to emphasize social aspects again.*

*Avoiding these issues is one possibility.
- *No. I am lucky enough to practice the way I want to practice and unencumbered by more traditional models of care.*
- *Definitely.*

Misc.
- *I concentrate more on quality of life. Five or six years ago I would try to gear more towards the overall health and well-being. Quality of life is important. With recent losses in my family I realize it plays a big role.*
- *I might go out on my own.*

Q: If so, how?

If so, when?

Q: If you had it to do all over again, would you become a doctor? Why? Why not?

One interviewee said, "I can't see myself doing anything else. This is who I am."

- *Yes.*
- *Yes.*
- *Yes.*
- *I probably would.*

- *Yes. I enjoy what I do. Sometimes people appreciate it, sometimes people don't. But at the end of the day when I go home I know that I have done the best for the patient to the best of my ability.*

- *Yes. It would be disrespectful to our profession. I like what I do except for certain things. It is a very satisfying profession. I tell my kids it is a good field. People will appreciate and that you are trying to get them better. New generation of physicians have a different mentality and different life. The people born here and raised here, they don't want to work like we do; they want 9-5 and be happy with a salary and travel and do other things that other people want to do. I don't see many gung ho and starting their own practices. I did that 8am -10pm for years and years. I don't know if it was worth it. I missed out a lot more than I gained personally, family wise kids wise. It is hard on my wife.*

- *I ask myself that regularly, that is a tough one. When the door is closed and I am with the patient I love it. I have made a good income but I work hard. So that was good. I found intellectually it was challenging and it was also good. I am not sure what else I would have done.*

- *I am going to say yes, except to say I am not sure that I would go through medical school and residency again. I like what I do. The whole training and time put in is certainly a lot of work compared to the financial rewards. It's a frustrating thing. People are looking at me like I am wealthy. I am comfortable and I am not hurting or starving. But most of my friends in business or law school are making a whole lot more money than I am. I find it frustrating at people looking at me like I am some rich guy.*

- *It's such a painful question. I would have gone to medical school and then gone to law school. Good consulting jobs. I wanted to take care of people. Can still take care of people. Even though I love what I do.*

- *Yes. I can't imagine doing anything else.*

- *Absolutely yes. I can't see myself doing anything else. This is who I am.*

- *Yes, except that I would have taken more business courses so that I understand business.*

- *I would. I love what I do. I always had a dream about finding what I wanted to do. At the end of the dream I realized I have it already.*

- *Absolutely.*

- *I would.*

- *I would because I really enjoy it. I couldn't see myself doing anything, else. I still consider myself lucky and privileged to be able to do it.*

- *Yes. So much of this interview is negative. Pluses more than minus. Satisfaction. Made a good living. In business for myself and did have to worry re being fired. It's upsetting to be fired.*

- *Yes. My son is becoming a doctor. I do know that he will not be the same doctor as I am. It's different.*

- *Yes. I can't think of anything else I'd be good at.*

- *Sure.*

- *Yes. I don't know what else I would do. I can't imagine doing anything different.*

- *Yes. My son is a doctor too.*

- *Yes. I embraced my inner Sherlock Holmes. It is cool. My spiritual journey is to be of service with the time that is have left on this earth. It is where the rubber meets the road. It gives my life meaning.*

- *Yes.*

- *Yes absolutely. I would probably run my own practice.*

- *Yes. One of my sons is a resident and so is his wife.*

- *Absolutely. This is awesome and I enjoy the social interactions with the patients.*

- *Yes.*

- *Because my vocation is to serve.*

- *YES. Definitely, I am good at it and I am not that good at much else and it is really fulfilling.*

- *Yes.*

- *Absolutely. I can't see myself being anything else. Including my children. It is a calling. I wouldn't discourage it or encourage it.*

- *Yes. I truly love what I do and I love to tell people that they are healthy and I will see you in a year.*

- *I would be a terrible businessman, I don't buy clothes. I wear a white coat.*

- *Yes.*

- *Yes. I enjoy. It makes me happy. I like coming to work and it makes me happy. I like who I am and what I do. There are some parts I don't like. I have a hobby. I have time for my kids. And some socializing. I like my kids to see that I do something that makes me happy. I take it and them seriously.*

- *I couldn't do anything else but be a doctor. I might have to rethink my specialty. I used to think I had to do primary care. Radiology, dermatology, anesthesiology, etc. I used to think that this didn't count as being a doctor.*

- *Definitely. I would absolutely do it all over again. Retired for 16 years. When I go to see my doctor, I run into old patients. Happy to be recognized. Happy to catch up. Patients are now parents themselves. One has grandchildren being raised with the same pieces of paper that I used to give out. Same papers for one-month visit through high school and college and now using them to raise children and grandchildren. I get hundreds of Christmas cards from old patients including pictures. We go to Maine from May to October and people come and visit us. They look us up and come.*

*Not sure or with a caveat.

- *Not sure. I have thought about it. My father worked so hard. If only I could have worked as hard as him. I'd be an accountant like my father. He did okay. No life on the line. Be an investment banker.*

- *I don't know. My husband has a horrible job, but medicine is better. But I'd do a specialty, not primary care. I might be a teacher. Summers off and time off with kids. Doctors you can basically work every second. This is what I am doing, so why look back.*

- *Yes but I would want to have the smarts to do it more efficiently and to be able to play the system.*

- *I'll tell you honestly this is a horrible question. Yes, because I always go home at night knowing that my days are never wasted and I am doing something right in the world. But my job has gotten harder and overregulated so I don't know if I will always be able to do it with abandon. The worries of how to navigate and survive in this world that it does sap the joy. I sometimes wonder what it is like in other fields that are not undergoing these changes. Fewer worries? More stable work/home life balance? Would another caring profession be better?*

- *Yes but not self-employed. The expense of a business and staff is almost impossible, to become an employee is difficult too and has to be examined. Training doctors has been the role financed by Medicare. Residencies and fellowships, Medicare. However, in the current system doctors are volunteering to teach. The funding is only through Medicare which is limited. The insurance companies get away without funding education although they are making huge demands on doctors. They expect the highest standards of care without helping to prepare. The hard working lose in this system. The ownership of the premiums – you really have to have ownership. If you lose one month of paying premiums. If you don't keep up, you are left with nothing. Most of them are publically traded and they are owned by stockholders. The citizens have to be stockholders. If the person paying the premium is willing to be an owner, they take responsibility. And they are partners. I have a stake in it. Residual value goes to premium payers not the insurance. Insurance has lost what it is. It used to be for major medical. Now it is that they should they pay for contraception.*

* Is it any wonder, given the lawsuits, the entitlement, the struggle to survive, the long intense hours, the debt, the cost to personal life, and the other stresses described by the doctor interviewees, that many of them would not choose to become a doctor again? Is it any surprise that according to the Association of American Medical Colleges that we have a frightening doctor shortage looming?

• *No. The regulations and other pressures that have been placed upon physicians have undermined the profession. The sacrifices, personal sacrifice to be a physician, it is not rewarded now. That is why I would not recommend another person becoming a physician. Mostly financially. Patients still thank me, so that is the same.*

* My interviewee was interrupted here by a page from the hospital about a very complicated patient.

Q: WOULD YOU RECOMMEND BEING A DOCTOR TO OTHER PEOPLE? WHY? WHY NOT?

* One said, "Yes if that's their passion." Another interviewee said, "It's a good way to live. You have a purpose."

• *Yes, but only if it is right for them.*

• *Only if you have a calling.*

• *Yes, but I would try and give them realistic expectations.*

• *Yes.*

• *Not as many as I would have early on. I think that to be a good doctor, the most important thing is you need to be smart. Be smart and be a nice, compassionate person. I see people who would be best off talking to a rock. This is a skill that you cannot learn. Yes, but I would be a little more concerned with that you need the people skills.*

- *Yes but only if they gave compassion and of course the stamina to go through training. Med school, residency, fellowship.*

- *Yes if that's their passion.*

- *If they have the same feelings I have then yes. It is very rewarding. Most of my friends are not docs. It never f elt genuine. Just taking me out for gold. My friends in business, their satisfaction revolved around someone getting screwed. That is not what medicine is all about. If someone has the right feeling, they will not make a lot of money so if that is what they want don't do it. You will be comfortable. You will work for a big group or a hospital. Solo docs will not be in the future. I like the business stuff, but most people don't and don't want have to deal with it.*

- *My son is a doctor. My daughter is a physical therapist, my other son just got into medical school.*

- *Yes. It is a really excellent field if you are curious and want to help people and have a problem solving mind. It is one of the few fields where you can do this. You have to be a little hard core. Today you do not have to give up your life. Lots of jobs, a family, being a woman is okay and it is not new.*

- *I still would. It is the greatest thing in the world to do.*

- *Oh sure, with full awareness that it is a lot of years of medical school and residency. The 50 years after that will more than compensate. Even during years of training are extremely satisfying — learning.*

- *Yes.*

- *I mentor people. You have to do what makes you happy. If taking care of people is what you enjoy do it. Not for prestige or money. There had to be nothing else that you want to do. You give up too much.*

- *Sure.*

- *Yes. But people for whom it would be suited.*

- *Yes. Once you have the feeling that this is what you want to do it is hard to think of anything else that is as rewarding and where there is as much knowledge about how our bodies work. This is exciting knowledge. If you understand that you have to the main thing has to be that you have compassion for people and want to help them, if you are doing it as prestige that is a stupid reason. For the money, if you want a comfortable life you will have that as a doctor, but it is not without cost. Financial. And the stresses and time issues. Holidays and family time. Go into it with eyes open. Love people and want to help and understand who we are, how our brains and bodies work. It's great. If you want a family you can have a flexible schedule in the right situation. Yes.*

- *Yes. It is still great. Can do a lot. Contribute a lot. Get involved in peoples' lives. I can see why young doctors would like to be employed and go home.*

- *It's a calling. It's not about money.*

- *You have to really really really want to be one. It does take a lot out of you. And there are some many impediments to having it be fulfilling today that were not there in the past. You have to be realistic. You can walk into the room and sit down from a total stranger and 30 or 40 minutes later it is intimate and there is nothing like it in other professions. It creates an awesome responsibility and you have to really realize that it is a huge responsibility and respect it or not take it on.*

- *Yes. It's important to follow your heart. If you want to be a doctor to help people, you should follow your heart.*

- *Only if there is nothing else that that you would rather do. You have to be totally devoted. This is not a career. It's a calling.*

- *Yes but with eyes wide open. I love what I do. But I would not want to head into it without knowing about the difficult road and the degree of compromise that you make and the uncertainty for the future. A profession that has high regard in society, but this is not the end all and be all, but it comes with a lot of sad times and disappointments. Watch other people who have chosen a different life have an easier time earlier in life. I show up late. I wasn't there at family events and I wanted to be there. You can't replace these things. Yes, but with eyes wide open. I would counsel people. Plus there are so many subspecialty areas.*

- *It's a good way to live. No mid-life crisis. You have a purpose.*

- *It depends on the person. Highly gratified, intellectually stimulating. Lots of good strokes from patients. But understand that you have to invest a lot of time and money to get there and there will be days that are incredibly stressful. It may also infringe on other things you want to do in life.*

- *If it makes you happy. Can't just do it for the money. If you don't like what you do then you are wasting your time. I want my kids to find something that they like.*

- *You have to be so sure. I could never tell anyone to try. You have to be honest about how difficult your life is.*

- *Sure if they have the burning desire to do it. They have different expectations. They want to be radiologists, dermatologists. They do not want to be me.*

- *Absolutely. Brainwashing the grandchildren to go into medicine. Smartest one. Accepted at Harvard and Princeton. Hoping for Princeton.*

- *Yes. I love being a doctor.*

* Some said, "No, I would not recommend being a doctor to other people." Sad, because although most of the interviewees are happy with their own lives as doctors, they would not recommend it to others. More evidence of the deterioration of our health care system. As one interviewee said, "But human nature and insurance companies are against us."Again, consider what the interviewees have explained about being a doctor and the looming doctor shortage.

- *I try and talk them out of it, but you can make a difference in people's life. But human nature and insurance companies are against us.*

- *No. I have told all of my children to not go into medicine. Who will take care of me when I am old and feeble? Medicine now is on the way down in terms of reimbursement and job satisfaction. I would like to think that this will improve and change but I don't know when that would be.*

- *No. I always tell people no.*

- *I tell people. If you can find anything else in life that will be as rewarding then you should do it. Be a physician assistant, if you just want to take care of people. No call. Have to be prepared to be under people. Can still make money.*

- *Not necessarily. Not everybody. I have probably mentored 100 doctors to medical school. It is not a matter of pull, it is a matter of mentoring. Five thousand applicants for 150 spots and there are a lot of well-qualified people out there. I will not do it on the basis of mother, father, or cousin. They come to my house and we talk for an hour especially doctors' children. Many of them don't want to go and they do not have the grades their father told me they have. I steer them to ancillary programs. Plus the reasons we have discussed are the reasons not to become a doctor. The biggest reason is the most highly overregulated profession in the world. Plus working at a job not a self-made practice. Reimbursement may or may not be adequate and it is extremely difficult to get it. It's a whole different system when you worked for yourself. I discourage a lot of people and encourage others who feel strongly.*

- *No. it is hard. My godson, he's 23. He was going to do it to give me a coffee break. I asked him if he was doing it for me don't do it. You are not compensated well for what you do. He is going to PT/OT. If you feel in your heart do it. Don't do it for money.*

- *No. I told my children that I do not want them going into medicine.*

- *I would not take the responsibility. I would let them decide themselves.*

- *No. I am being forced to think of medicine as a business and spending a half million on getting training has a poor return.*

- *I am not sure that I would become a doctor if I had it to do over again. I like what I do. I like helping people and having a positive impact in healthcare and lives, but it is a long road to become a doctor. 4.4.4. It can be very stressful. It is a challenging career. It is really challenging every day. Some of the things that I was talking about. I would not recommend it to my children. Because society, as it is currently constructed, does not recognize the value (not financially) of being a doctor. For all those years of training, they could train for something else, have less stress, and less student loans.*

Q: IS TRAINING TO BE A DOCTOR DIFFERENT NOW?

* One important way is that duty hours are restricted. This came to be as a result of the Libby Zion case in New York City in 1984. The somewhat controversial details of her situation are beyond the scope of this book. However, her family believed her death to be caused, at least in part, by overworked resident physicians. The result was that resident physicians, unlike attending or practicing physicians, are restricted in the amount of hours that they can work. This is mostly seen by the doctor interviewees as a negative for the patients. One doctor interviewee said, "It is more like shift work. Like a job. There is a reason they called us residents. It was more like life commitment." Another doctor said, "It was your patient until they went home. You don't hand the patients off to someone else." I got other answers like, "They are not being taught to think. They are being trained to order tests." And, "Young residents are experts in defensive medicine, rather than the real issues." The younger doctors are also not prepared for the "typical day or week" demands of practice, as they were described previously by the more experienced doctor interviewees.

• *Restricted hours. We didn't have them and it prepares you better. Residents have unrealistic expectations of what medicine is. Commitment to patients is different. They want to do 9-5. Everyone is looking for bigger groups. It's less personal. Not an intimate relationship that once was there between a patient and doctor.*

- *They don't work as hard as I did. I worked 120 hours per week. They have no idea what is scut work. We drew blood etc. They don't look at urine or cell counts. We made slides. No transport service, i.e. for x-rays. Had to get them approved. Had to find a wheel chair or a stretcher. Had to take things to the lab ourselves. I had to make friends with them to get labs run. I worked a lot harder. We had to get along with the older attendings. The art of sitting and talking to people is a lost art. No one does that any more. May not need a CT scan or a blood count. Just sit and listen. The personal care that people had is not there. My grandmother has horrible arthritis. My parents took her to a star. She didn't like him. No personal contact. This is why you go into medicine, not to order tests.*

- *It's easier. There are limits on hours. My dad worked 120 hours a week in the Bronx. I worked 36 hours in a row and was on call every third night. A little easier. It is changing with the times. It's not good for people to do it anyway. A lot of fellows pick something easier.*

- *The same but with new rules about hours it is changing. When I was in training, even though we were post call we made sure that the patient was stable before we leftj. Now because of the 80 hour rules have to leave post call so I am not sure that they are developing the sense of belonging to patients which is important.*

- *Yes I think that it is. The residency program that I did was way different than what they are doing now. So much push to limit the hours and they are caped with patients. When I was a resident whatever walked in the door you took. If you got no sleep. We would regularly work 36 hours. Now they come in and they see the patient and go home at 4 or 5. It is supposed to contribute to better patient safely. I don't know.*

When you are exhausted you make more mistakes but there was always somebody above you. An attending. Even the nurses, they aren't going to do something that is really bad By working that way in a constant state of sleep deprivation the stuff became innate and you could make decisions almost without thinking. I would wake up and check and it was always the right thing to do. You've got to be able to do it and that is important and following the patient through the hospitalization was important. It was your patient until they went home. You don't hand the patients off to someone. The hospitalists are going to burn out. Like ER doctors. You can't do that for 25 years. But shift work is the same way it is. You will come in, punch your clock and go home. No compassion.

- *Now it is 9-5. They don't have to think on their feet. A lot of this has to be immediate and automatic. They want you to deal with emergencies and do it. You learn how to deal with people. That weeded out the bad doctors. Now you can only have a certain number of hours then they give them over to the attending doctors. You see the difference in the quality for the residents. It's sad.*

- *We don't do the 36 hours straight. The younger doctors don't have the commitment. They want 9-5, a retirement plan, no calls.*

- *Yes. It's all shift work.*

- *It is not as hard core. You were in the hospital for 90 hour weeks and I ran the show. One hundred patients in the ER, a disaster and a code. You learn how to manage crises and now there are so many restrictions on the hours it impedes their training in the younger years. Too much supervision, i.e. for a Tylenol. They never see the whole picture. I was with the patient from the beginning to the end. It let me be a good doctor today. Today you need a fellowship. They are sleeping more and they are not learning as much. They are not forced to make decisions. Its helicopter training. You learn how to make decisions when you are on your own. The younger doctors. A different breed. They are a little bit more, they expect that they do not have to work. If time is up, they leave, in the old days you did not leave until you were done. This is a vocation and a calling and requires sacrifice. Not so much of that now. They rely on digital. They Google things on rounds. They don't do the research. The answers come too easily and you do not absorb it quite as much.*

- *Have to defend yourself and be involved politically. Yes. It is desensitization. The doctor today is assumed to be compliant doctor. Fee for service is looked down on. Compliant means: understands the role of the hospital. They have no idea what it is like to meet payroll and run a business. They are not trained. When they come here they get trained. Eighty percent work for hospitals now and when I graduated it was 20 percent. Now they just want to get a salary and go home.*

- *Fewer hours on call.*

- *Easier. A lot of laws now. Like the hours. They ask re hours and vacation. Everyone wants to work less for the same money. Evaluating the practice, is that we count them as .75 if they are less than 45 years old.*

- *They are not being taught to think. They are being trained to order tests.*

- *Young residents are experts in defensive medicine, rather than the real issues.*

- *Very different. The government screwed it up. Eighty-hour work week. The patient who died had psychiatric problems and didn't tell the doctors what meds she was on. When I was a resident I was responsible for patients. Even when I left, it was mine. You took the patient home. Responsibility. Now you are a shift worker and you may never see that patient for days. Major unintended consequences. Hospitalist. The doc who knows you doesn't go to the hospital. You are a lot less human.*

- *It is longer now and it was too long then. Subspecialty training. Mine was 13 years. Now add two more years of fellowship it is too long and most of what you learn you forget except what you still use.*

- *The work hour restrictions. Good and bad side effects. It has really decreased the hours of call that residents have to do. But at the same time it decreases their exposure to patients. It's very difficult for training to make sure that the residents get the same quality training and exposure that I had. I took care of the patient and I stayed until the patient was safe and it was okay for me to leave. I didn't walk out.*

- *It is my understanding, a lot. I don't teach at the medical school level to know. A couple of major areas. There are restrictions on work hours. Pros and cons. Pro-the doctor is more awake. Con-it sets up a system of hand-off. Nobody is in charge of a patient. Lack of sleep of deprivation goes away after training. A discord. The doctors are still in practice hiring younger doctors with stricter work hours. They feel that the younger generation is taught to be lazy. Other reality- if you have never had to do work at night what happens when your patients call in the middle of the night. Can't say it's not my patient. There was abuse, but we swung the opposite way. A couple of the guys in my department of who will take care of them when old. They don't want the younger ones taking care of them. We facilitate the lazy ones and it is harder to weed them out and keep looking for the good ones.*

- *It is more like shift work. Like a job. There is a reason they called us residents. It was more like life commitment.*

- *Less time spent in residency. Due to residency has restricted hours.*

- *Cut the hours 9-5. I hope that enough people with a serious work ethic can give the same continuity of care. If they breed doctors who have no interest in what happens to you after 5, that's not good. They should make the residencies longer. Need the same type of exposure. Certain things only happen at night. More time to sleep doesn't mean that they sleep or read. Economics can be a source of stress.*

- *Bell commission laws — not allowed to work more than 30 hours in a row. A lot of simulations that the patients go through now. It's a lot more controlled environment. More availability of patient centered discussions, how to talk to patients and how to interview them. It is improving slowly.*

- *Yes, because of all the bureaucratic red tape that you have to know that goes with it.*

* There are some clinical differences and some positives in current training.

- *No, but they are getting better with social and emotional stuff.*

- *Yes, it is. They are conscious of the fact that physicians do not know how to talk to people and there are courses, are geared towards how you talk to a patient.*

- *It's so different. They have to write papers and do research. They are more driven to the specialties than to primary care.*

- *Much different. It is very advanced. It is much more clinically oriented today which is good. They have a lot more opportunities with robotic medicine and the opportunity to do hands on and earlier on. They get clinical work their first year.*

- *I don't know. I don't think so. I deal with the students. The body is the body. The tests and information are on line. The information is pretty much the same. How you acquire if is different. Pops ups about what meds people are on and the interactions. I have been encouraged by the docs who come through. I do their first clinical course. Freshman year. They have just been studying the books and they are taking the courses in physical diagnosis. They follow me to see that is like with a doctor patient for real. Don't live them, don't hate them, just treat them. Do what you have to do. A mentor told me this.*

- *I don't teach. It is not a strength. They seem eager. You are getting more people who want to do it for the right reasons than in the past. In the past people went into it for money and prestige and their parents wanted them to do it.*

- *More information and techniques. They are really bright. They know a lot more. They won't be in private practice. Salaried position but better hours. They will be home more. I always tried to make my kids games. I have two woman partners. They want to be home too. No one says at the end if their life I wish I worked more. Rather be with family.*

- *More emphasis on proficiency that knowledge. Now you have to determine that you actually can do something. Not just understand it.*

- *Why don't you interview them? How would I know? The training is quite different. The basic science is the same. The science is compressed. They have more clinical time. They use the computer naturally and exclusively. They will be much more practice guideline oriented. But the basic idea of humanism and taking care of patients has not changed. One cousin teaches it. We never were taught.*

Misc

- *Most definitely.*

- *I presume so. Too far away from academia to answer that question.*

- *Yes.*

- *More multicultural and with language differences. I had a more select group of people more like my background than now. Different backgrounds and expectations.*

*Technology makes it different.

- *Computer stuff. They are better at it.*

- *Yes. EMR's. The internet. Patients come in and know information. The older docs don't like it that the younger docs leave early. They are doing it differently. I don't think that they are worse. The new generation will be able to balance life better and do things with their families and friends. It was better for me not to be home. I would have been a doting mom. So by the time I got home, they already had their bruises. Don't be home so that my kids could learn scary things.*

- *I believe so. I do not have a direct hand in it. Major resources available, Ie internet to enrich the capacity of training and other technologies.*

Q: ARE THE YOUNGER DOCTORS DIFFERENT NOW?

* Some of the differences are attributed to reduced duty hours. Managed care makes a negative contribution as well.

• *Yes, it may be better for the younger doctors because they can spend more time with their families, but it is not for the better for patients. They are shift workers.*

• *They come out looking for a 9-5 job. Managed care has created this idea that you can work 9-5 and don't have to build a practice and invest money. They attract a different kind of physician. Women are in medicine now and they can take time off for maternity leave, which was very difficult before. And a diversion of talented people away from medicine. It is lessprestigious than in the past. It has been deflated a little bit.*

• *Yes, they are more expecting to not work the hours that I work. I am looking for an associate. No one is going to work my hours. They don't want to work as hard because of their training. They didn't work so hard.*

• *When I started you put your time in and tried to become a partner. You knew you would work hard. You could not have $250K to buy into your share, so it was taken out in sweat and salary. The young doctors want it right away. So they take jobs with high salary and are almost not interested in owning practices, urgi-cares etc.*

• *They want a job and quality of life verses someone who is really dedicated. We are not bankers. You cannot squelch that drive and bring doctors to the top.*

• *The system is going to draw in a different type of physicians in general. Potentially not the cream of the crop. Many people went into medicine to care for people but not have to*

*worry about income. Work hard, care for people, but not
have to worry about money. That doesn't exist. On the other
hand you can now work for a health care system, make less
money, and be out at a certain time and not worry when you
leave. Someone else will take care of it. The younger doctors
still want the same things. They want to take care of people,
be compassionate, help people and have relationships with
the people. The new grads. The ones that are intermediate
to me in their late 30s or 40s, they feel that they have been
cheated. They had a vision and a promise of what they would
be and their whole world crumbled. That leads sometimes
to bad behavior. When you don't have to worry about income
and money and try to do what is right and sometimes the
behavior changes. What you expected what you would have
is taken away and you have to generate income in ways that
you may have not needed to do previously. See more patients
for a shorter period of time. Order more tests to develop more
income. Maybe setting up more businesses to have people
work under you that you cannot quality assure now.
Everything is based upon generating income. You didn't
have an income problem in the past. I want to clarify that
even in the old days, people did well and people still wanted
more. The system has changed so that the government and
the insurance companies are trying to restrict, control,
follow and manage, that they have built an infrastructure of
red tape that now has the physical hurdles though to game
the system. How do you play the game and do the best that
you can in the system? The note is the biggest joke, so they
set up the EMR and criteria, have to go from A to Z and all
people do is duplicate the note. It is still the last paragraph
that tells what the patient needs to get the appropriate
amount of charge for the time that you have given. They,*

the government and the insurances, have gone too far to the right and have placed the wedge. They missed the boat, how to give good patient care and save costs. They are paying other people to monitor others activities and those people get around it. It will come back, but they have missed the boat for now. They have set up barriers to take care of the people properly. The way that press portrays it is that the doctors just want to grab money. Doctors are afraid of getting sued. I do not have that issue fortunately. I never focus on getting sued. At least half of the doctors are concerned with lawsuits. This is another reason for why physicians over order. They are so paranoid and this is what they focus on. When you are afraid of something and you keep trying not to get into trouble you get into trouble. This was one thing I don't worry about. If I practice good medicine, I will be okay. But, I could be unlucky, be in the wrong place at the wrong time.

- *Millennials. They are all so entitled. They think that they don't have to work and 80 hours per week is a problem. The mistakes I made in medical training were not due to sleep deprivation. Mistakes were due to not enough help or fear to ask for help. Lack of guidance. Plus you need to learn how to take care of people when you are tired. When they come out into practice, they don't know how to do it. One doctor accidentally made a mistake with a baby, which then required surgery, and the doctor followed the ambulance in a rainstorm to my office and they did not sue. The resident in this case was at home. I told her that she hurt her patient and should be present. THIS IS YOUR PATIENT AND YOU ARE RESPONSIBLE FOR IT.*

- *Yes. Because of everything we have talked about.*

- *Yes. I think of the medical students that come through my office. Smart. Super-smart. But I think there is a definite more of a 9 to 5 attitude. I could be wrong. But there is a more 9 to 5 attitude from what I see. It doesn't happen often that people graduate school and open practice. More and more are employed and it is more shift work. You are not 24/7 on. I see how it would be attractive. That's where it's going. A hospitalist gets off at 7 and that's it, they are done. They are not fielding phone calls and things like that.*

- *They seem more mechanized to me. I am not around a lot of them. But they seem more routine, more coming out to get an 8-5 job.*

- *I don't know enough of them. I do get a sense however that the changes in healthcare have selected for a different type of doctor. It used to be more individualistic. Long range develop type and practice. Didn't have to worry so much about being efficient. You could make mistakes and they are not fatal. They have to face the reality that they are going to be part of a group and the business aspects will not be in their control. Simpler lives in some respects. Practice medicine and have nothing to do with the business and organization aspects of running a practice.*

- *Better hours in residency. That is a good thing. There is not a benefit to being sleep deprived, stay up all night, sleep away from your family. You don't have to suffer that much to be a great doctor. I don't know enough about them to answer the other questions.*

- *Yes. They are shift workers. They want to finish their shift and go home. The mentality is to finish their shift and go home. JCAHO regulations – they can only work a certain hours of work.*

- *Yes, because of shifts.*

- *Yes they are coming into a world of practice now that is going to make them not individual entrepreneurs anymore. They all join groups. Their expectations for reimbursement are higher than what we started out building a practice from nothing. They are coming out with more debt. They will never be able to take on the overhead. So their expectations are different. Salary, discreet hours and very light call schedule.*

- *Yes. Because the teaching is more fragmented. There is no holistic approach as we had in the past. They do not have the patients experience because of bureaucratic limitations they are not allowed to practice on patients and do procedures.*

- *They are different. Not the same hours. They work less hours. It is mandated. They have no choice. Don't think it's fair to say that they do not have the same work ethic. It does not give them the same opportunity to be immersed in medicine. It may make them less tired and less stressed but I don't think that it will make them better doctors. They also do not have the same autonomy as early as we had it. They are excessively supervised which I think limits their decision making abilities.*

- *Yes. Their expectations are not to enter practice but to enter a hospital or corporation. 50-60 percent of them do so.*

- *No doubt about it. Good and bad. They are interested in their own lifestyles. They try to be more available for their own families. Doctors in my generation neglected their ow families because they were so busy. Now people want a schedule that allows them to be better parents than we were.*

- *Duty hours. The residents in training have always worked long hours. Correctly the regulating bodies have focused on limiting the hours, which is a good thing. It is a positive, in addition to over stressing the doctors in training as well as considering the patients. Duty hours and proper supervision are good. But the concern that I have now is that they are coming into me with a shift work mentality. May be a good coping mechanism for them for dealing with stressors , but the concern is will they have the same sense of follow- through, ability, and caring. By in large, most of them have it. But I see a gradual shifting in there. My question is who is going to then take care of me down the road? Is it going to be a doc who has that sense of caring and follow- through or not? Not just the shift work mentality, but experience. As the duty hours have changed, the residents are required to do more paperwork. Case logs, online surveys to the regulation organizations, all of this is pulling them away from the bedside and further developing their skills and confidence. We have to keep an eye on this over time – the profession and society. I am comforted to see that so many of the students and residents do have a sense of caring and dedication to the patients. A strong sense. I am encouraged but I am concerned that the system will beat them down.*

- *Different opportunities, but different expectations.*
- *They are 9 to 5. No weekends or holidays. Not like us.*

* No, the younger doctors are not different.
- *No they are still starry eyed and they are going to save the world. They rejuvenate the office.*
- *I don't think so. But, they are equally concerned on making a living and spending time with family.*
- *I don't think so.*

- *They can be just as idealistic and caring but they have a different expectation of their schedule. They definitely want to have a life. And they do not have the entrepreneurial spirit to run a practice.*

Misc

- *I don't know. But I think that it should be. I think medical school should be three years, not four. The costs of medical school has skyrocketed and we need to see that cost under control and this is the only way to do it. I think that a lot of the specialty learning could be provided to physicians as they enter specialty that requires that additional training.*
- *Yes and no. So many factions in America. Shifts start and we are not aware of them happening.*
- *Some are and some aren't. Luck of the draw.*

Q: IF SO, HOW?
DO THEY HAVE ANYTHING THAT YOU DIDN'T HAVE?
ARE THEY MISSING SOMETHING THAT YOU HAD?

* They have the advantage of technology.

- *They have computers. I had to remember everything. They can check and see if I am BSing them.*
- *They do have better skills with technology. But I didn't have it when I came out and I am good with technology. You don't need journals and textbooks and you don't need it now, it is immediately available. I would call the library to do a search and I would get it a week later. More burdensome. That is great. They are missing the ability to spend more time with patients and to get to know them which markedly improves the doctor-patient relationship. They are in and out. Their time constraints are different.*

- *The training is not different, they are not different. The system is different. They have better computer skills.*

- *Are they missing something that you had? Computers. We had to run down to the lab. They are missing the in the trenches work that we did but they have more tools.*

- *Are they missing something that you had? Not yet. They are going to have pocket ultrasounds for diagnosis. Stethoscopes will go out of vogue.*

- *They have the internet. They don't have to go to the library and look everything up. The technology today and the access to information is so superior to what it was. That is a big advantage. And the amount of information that you have to access.*

- *Technology.*

- *They are better at team work than we are. They are much more proficient at computers and accessing information.*

- *They have a better understanding of the electronic aspects of medicine. Their medical school bills might be their biggest source of stress, but I don't know.*

* They are missing certain aspects of training that often leads to a different work ethic.

- *More training in the non-medical aspects of medicine. They are missing the pleasure of being on call 36 hours straight and being on call every second, third night. Now there are strict limits of hours per week and how long. They are better rested. The training is longer so they get it.*

- *I came from a mentality that you have to work hard and teach yourself things. Nowadays there is a lot of spoon feeding. They are not as proactive and rely on other things and other people to help them out.*

- *More sense of entitlement and a sense of they won't work as long and as hard. They don't have the time commitments.*
- *They have debt. They seem like they are there for the right reason. I am sure that some of them are there because their parents told them to be doctors. These will not be good docs.*
- *They are missing a different work ethic. It's not quite the same.*
- *They have a personal life.*
- *They have more time. I had better training. I did not worry about the stress.*
- *No. I hope that they understand when they come into practice that they will be expected to take care of an emergency at 3 in the morning even if you are tired.*
- *Yes. They have a more realistic view of cost benefit. Things cost money so don't just go down a path to theoretically run people through some tests. More efficient. Missing – gung ho, total abandon, this is my patient and I am not going to walk out until everything is set, versus my residency program will be shut down if I stay any longer.*
- *They are only missing the desire to be a primary care doc.*
- *A winning lottery ticket. My innocence.*
- *I don't think so. It still takes the same drive, guts and ignorance to do it.*

Misc

- *I went to a great medical school. I don't know. I don't interact with them much. People here appreciate what you do for them as opposed to where I live.*
- *Both.*

- *Not answerable.*

- *I can't give a negative answer here. No to my recollection. I see them at conferences and we talk and I never say something like that.*

- *No. No.*

Q: **WHAT IS THEIR BIGGEST SOURCE OF STRESS?**

* Finances are a big source of stress. Doctors come out of medical school in debt. The average debt is around $225,000. Compare that to a salary of less than $200,000 per year for a primary care doctor. Now imagine trying to get a mortgage, feed and clothe your children, pay living expenses, and all of the other responsibilities of adulthood, with that kind of debt. Never mind working the hours that my interviewees described in an earlier chapter of this book. It would be definitely stressful.

- *Financial and cost of education.*

- *Their loans. And the job market. They don't have the same opportunities. Everyone wants to be in their area. They get paid less here. Oversaturation. They don't have the choice to pick their job.*

- *Money and the legislative and professional mandates, part of which are created by government and insurance companies and their own professional organizations.*

- *Their financial situation. It will be years before they can get a mortgage. They are so under water.*

- *Debt. Incomes are coming down as incomes for insurance companies go up. The taxes are worse and the income is worse and the debt is worse.*

- *The cost of education.*

- *The financial burden to become a doctor.*

- *Financial. That is their world.*

- *They are better off in at least they have a job, but they graduate with debt. They don't know where their future is heading. After a while it's all behind you so it doesn't matter. My kids who are doctors will have a great life but they have to figure out how to have a family life. They will do okay economically but they need to be able to balance their lives.*

* So is time. The interviewees described their work schedules earlier in this book.

- *They all complain about how hard they work and not enough sleep. Are you kidding me?*

- *They don't handle stress as well as we did. They break down and cry and life gets in the way. We did not have a life. We waited. So they have more stresses because they have a life. We did residency for three years.*

- *Time restraints. Documentation. Office. Hospital. Trying to do the best you can wherever you go.*

- *They haven't quite gotten the fact that they are not going to have the same amount of free time and liberty that they would have had otherwise. That is stressful. They are book smarter than we were. But they have less common sense.*

- *Their lifestyle. They want a good one.*

* As always, there are clinical stresses.

- *The difficult diagnostic problem, when you want to make sure that you are not missing something and are on the right track with a problem. You have to work at it. Review some literature or refer the patient to a major specialty center. The tough management of tough problems. Managed care. Still the most important stress is the demands of taking care of a complex patient.*

- *Same as us. Being on call. Handling patients post call but as the years go by you learned that those are the times that you gain the most knowledge and experience because you are managing the patients.*

- *Getting into a specialty.*

- *Going out into practice they will have to deal with the same mandates and requirements that I have to deal with now. They should learn from other doctors in practice. Take as many courses in economics and legal aspects of medicine as they can. Many of these courses are offered by our specialty societies.*

- *In this difficult economy finding a good practice position and what to choose. They stress about some of the same things I stressed about. Impressing their trainers so that they can advance to good training places. Work life balance and raising families.*

- *In medical school it was knowing that you could study, bust your ass and work as hard as you can and still fail a test, then be on the chopping block. But I loved medical school.*

- *Loans and learning to cope with what we talked about isn't easy it is not for everyone. Just because you are smart and did well on the MCAPS doesn't mean that you can do well with this other stuff.*

* Or both.
- *Passing tests and financial issues.*
- *Financial uncertainty and home verses work balance.*

Misc
- *I don't want to worry about money. I just want to be a doctor.*

- *Not knowing the future.*
- *I don't know.*
- *They don't talk to me. We don't get into those details. We socialize or talk about memory of old cases.*
- *I don't know.*
- *I couldn't say.*

Q: WHAT WOULD YOU LIKE TO TELL THEM?

- *Help each other out. Listen to the patient. The patient will usually tell you what is wrong with them.*
- *Retire early. Communists and socialists: Don't F it up.*
- *Don't forget your family. If people go into it for money it's not going to bring them happiness. They have to love what they do or they will burn out and crash. Balance life and try to do what you can at work.*
- *It's worth it.*
- *Nothing. Because if they are going into medicine for the right reason, they love people and the science. They have to take the good with the bad and change medicine. You don't not go into a profession that you love because of a governmental system that has made it so difficult. Some people don't go into medicine because of the money. They can't reach their dream. It may be multiple dreams, they can't get the whole package. I wouldn't tell them that. You need to do what you love to do each day.*
- *To grow up.*
- *It's a great life. Great way to make a living and be part of a community.*
- *They need to be encouraged and need to go into primary care. By making them and the patients independent. The*

independent patient is the only one where the diagnosis is not known. In New York if you are depressed they can come in and take your gun. Are you going to open up to your doctor? Or are you going to talk about feeling suicidal?

- *Go into medicine and get involved in people's lives.*
- *Medicine is a profession that doesn't end at 5:00.*
- *The importance of humanism.*
- *Nothing. It is changing. I don't know what to tell them. The practice of health care is changing. Don't get so freaked out about a malpractice case. It's not about bad care, it's about bad outcomes and you are not responsible for bad outcomes.*
- *Don't expect the practice of medicine what your dad's and grandpa's was. But be realistic and enjoy it; it is still pretty special.*
- *The sad fact is that I don't tell them anything right now. I don't have a road map for them that is useful. Develop a skill set that is as sub-specialized and profound so that you can have a skill that others don't have so that you can remain viable.*
- *If Obama called me. Should not be profit. I paid for my kids' medical school. Train for five or six years after medical school. Why do that if not making a fair amount of money. But don't want them to own a surgi center, x-ray facilities, PT services. Don't want them to have those things, although they would make a fortune. Pay doctors well, but shouldn't incentive them to do more. The Accountable Care Organizations are bankrupting our country. Take the profit out and pay doctors a good salary. Make sure that families own part of the system and they have to pay for part of the system. Have a higher deductible. Have people pay part of it. Only practice medicine that is recommended by the*

Academy of Medicine. Recommendations for certain things. If a drug company wants to introduce a drug. Use drugs that are most effective. Only introduce drugs that are more effective and have evidence that it will work. And make the person live longer. Heath care has to be rationed. Have a budget. My family has a budget and there is no evidence that we have a better success than other countries. Cost of making drugs and have to show the results of their studies. All of them. Make the patients pay part of their care. Prilosec and Nexium and other drugs and there is no difference. They tweak it a bit. It should be against the law. This is just another way to hold on to the patient. We should only do tests that make people better. In medical school we were taught to make diagnosis with no thought of the cost. We should be graded on getting people better and the cost of care too. This is the real world. The insurance companies tell me how I am doing economically. Hospitals want to throw off people who do too many expensive procedures, unless you can prove that your survival rate is higher. You have to explain why that is. My death rates are high because my patients are older. You can't rank doctors. Patients are all different. Cookbook therapy doesn't work. You have to pick and choose what to treat with older patients or those on too many meds. What is the most important disease? That is part of medical judgment. When do you choose to treat something or not, I.e. if someone is dying? It doesn't make any sense. Patients have to understand that there are some economic constraints that have to be applied. Can't just be admitted to the hospital anymore. Patients get pissed with high co-pays. The unions don't want to pay more. Baby boomers are going to destroy the generations afterwards. Somebody else has to get on the tennis court. People believe that there is a breakthrough and you can live forever. If you live a full life and make it to 90 or 100 its over. What is quality of life? I don't know, but I know it when I see it. And change the malpractice system They threaten you. Extortion letters, i.e. sue for criminal negligence because malpractice won't pay it, so that they ask for money not to sue.

• *Nothing.*

Q: What do they need that they don't have?

* Experience. They don't have enough time with patients. Again, because of duty hours and insurance problems.

• *Brains. Experience.*

• *Guidance. When I was at that stage I had no one to tell me what to do when I got out and what to do and what to expect about how medicine will change or they will be in for a big shock and make a lot mistakes as they go along. It takes its toll on you. So be ready for that.*

* More time and skill with patients.

• *They need to work at people skills. It is damaging. People skills require time, you have to spend time with the patients. Because of the way the system is set up there is less face time. You need to be able to look at patients to see the impact on a patient. Body language is an important diagnostic feature. You need to look at this stuff.*

• *They need to have a sense of responsibility and obligation to their patients.*

• *They need more mentoring and hands on training. No virtual anatomy. They don't even touch the corpse so they need hands on training for the physical.*

- *They need more time with patients and less with papers and computers.*
- *Preparedness for sleep deprivation and may not have a life that is as good as what they had in training. They will have the opposite of what we had.*
- *I don't think that they have quite the same sense of personal responsibility because they are so good at team work. They are so good at teamwork that defuses responsibility. We are better at saying I am responsible and I am not going home until the last patient is seen. We are not so good at team work.*

* Less financial stress
- *They have everything that I had. Maybe. I didn't have the bills that they have. My education was very inexpensive. My son's education is $60,000 for medical school. They have the internet.*
- *Less debt.*

Misc.
- *Ask them. I don't see them in practice. I see them at conference. We are all pretty equal.*

Q: WHAT NEEDS TO CHANGE?

* The very basics of the healthcare system need to change.

- *Reimbursements. The amount of money that is being wasted. Multiple trips to ER, multiple scans, etc. the way the residents are being trained. To rely on imaging, not clinical judgment and physical exam. Over prescription of imaging studies. Costs more money.*
- *Get rid of Obama. Be intelligent and ask questions.*
- *It would be nice to be compensated better so that you don't have to see so many people. Independent. Running a*

company. Salaries and overhead. It would be great to be able to spend a half hour with every visit but you can't make it that way.

- *Solve the problem, a two health care system income plus socialized medicine for the rest of the people. We are going to have the haves and the have nots.*

- *We need to get away from shift work in medical training. If hospitals didn't depend on residents to fill the labor gaps and instead commit residents to learning actual skills. Sometimes we used to clean rooms so we would do it as residents. They wanted us to do all of this labor. Hire a NP or a PA for overnight not residents rather than using the 80 hours for it. On night float you aren't learning. Coverage is not learning.*

- *The entire system of funding. There should be some consideration for physicians to get rid of some of these debts, either by scholarship debt relief it they stay within the stare for a certain number of years. Ie work in underserved areas. The federal government already has that. We are trying to get it into the state. This extraordinary system of maintaining your licensure and certification, which is overdone and has no proven benefit. Unnecessarily burdensome and abusive.*

- *I can't see things from the way I was. If you talked to omeone who worked 24 hours a day and had no one to sign out to.*

- *We need privacy. We need government that really respects freedom.*

- *Leave them alone and let them learn. Don't have all of the regulations.*

- *The lack of consistency in health care policy. The inconsistency of reimbursement to different physicians. We need to see a change in the way physicians are compensated. It should not be about who has the best relationship with the payers. It should be based on outcomes and years for practice. Electronic health medical records should be able to communicate with each other from practice to practice. We should see an evolution to telemedicine.*

- *Malpractice reform.*

- *It is not going to change very fast. It is like turning an ocean liner. What needs to be empathized and some of the medical schools are doing it more is they have to emphasize the compassion side more. The communication skills. The science has been primarily skills and when they come out they find that not everything is as straightforward. Listen to the patient. If they tell you something that doesn't make sense take a moment to think that it is you not them. Out of medical school too much arrogance to think that is possible.*

- *The whole system needs to be torn down. Politicians and lawyers need to get out of interfering with medicine. Medicine cannot be a one glove fit all profession. They are different tiers of medicine. People who can afford insurance. There should be no limitations on patients on who they can see, when they can see or where they can go to get treatment. Have high deductible or catastrophic. People who cannot afford it can go to clinics. Nothing is fair. Connected with medical schools and hospitals and you get good care. People are training there. Life is not fair.*

- *Over protectiveness of the training institutions. Setting up some barriers to work related stress and overwork, but removing the restrictions on work hours so not restrictive.*

- *Triangulation with insurance companies for lawsuits. Same thing with patient care. When you give somebody something for free, that is exactly how they value it. It needs to go back to the patients keeping themselves well, not the doctor. Then it is the doctor's fault.*

* Time with patients

• *More personal interaction.*

• *Time. They need more time with their patients.*

• *They need to get more patient interaction experience and responsibility.*

• *In my old office they are hiring more young pediatricians who work half time so that their schedules can accomplish their family needs. It's good. More women than men now going into my specialty.*

Q: **How can that be accomplished?**

• *I don't know. If they change the whole system to a one payer system, there might be some improvement.*

• *If you are going to cause medicine to become socialized then go the whole way. Any other country the education is paid for.*

• *Limit liability so that you don't have to over test. Take the incentives away for over utilizing the system. Double edged sword. People will leave, unless people are paid what is appropriate for the time they put in they will leave or have crappy medicine. The computer system has to be user friendly clinically pertinent and not meet the needs of engineers and people who don't have any experience clinically. Things will change in 10 years.*

• *Hard work and persistence. First through the professional associations have allowed the legislative and the insurance companies to use this stuff against them.*

- *Leadership in organized medicine which is sorely lacking.*

- *Go back to family doctors. We are overly specialized. Pressed into specializations because they cannot make a living as family doc. Lack of primary care doc prevents good care. Breaks a patient into parts to fix the broken parts. We need holistic medicine again where 99 percent of what you have the internist can take care of.*

Q: WHAT IS/ARE THE BIGGEST UNRESOLVED ISSUE(S) IN MEDICINE? WHY IS THIS SO HARD TO UNDERSTAND?

- *We have a bizarre system. How we pay for it, litigate it, regulate it etc. We don't need giant profit-seeking insurance companies in the middle of it to second guess what we do. On the other hand is the government, the way to regulate it. We are right in the middle of what the patients want and need and what the system is willing and is going to pay for something. If I do something I will be denied, if I don't do it I will be sued. Other players are ready to second guess you.*

- *How to pay us. I am working on committees to work on guidelines. Computers can help us zero in on patients who need us the most.*

- *Preventive care. Addressing preventative issues.*

- *How to improve quality of care while making sure that everyone has decent and affordable insurance. A chain of bureaucracy and who will cover what and whether you will get what you need. Have to spend money for care. As soon as people come down on the insurance companies and tell them to stop making billions of dollars. The patient is last. The insurance companies- you cannot fight with them. Calls about a prescription. I might as well not write the prescription. I have some CEO telling me what to prescribe. There are people who are freeloaders and live off our system; others are people who work all day and cannot afford insurance. Blue collar and working hard, there is something wrong with this whole system. People who need medicines cannot have them it. People who don't take care of themselves and get Medicaid and get everything for free. People who live off our system and our tax dollars and they don't work a single day. And there are patients who I see and cannot afford medicines and need them. These other patients can get medication for free and they don't take it anyway. Huge co-pays. Lots of unresolved issues. The biggest one is long term care. It is a huge problem. Nursing homes are horrible and people live longer. No quality of care in nursing homes. The regulations are not there and the quality of care is not there. So what will people do? Problems with paperwork and ambulances. The patients who need it can't get it. I can't lie for people.*

- *The economics of universal access care in a world of incredibly expensive medicine.*

- *It is so complicated. The insurance needs to be unified and simplified. It is too complicated. The whole process needs to be simplified. One payer system.*

- *A big thing called social medicine that is somewhat lacking. Doctors are always in a rush and sometimes we miss out on talking to the patient about their social issues. What is going on at home, do they have someone to talk to? Should be a branch called social medicine. We do have social workers in the hospital but an MD with that specialization.*

- *How to provide good healthcare to an entire population in an affordable fashion. That is very difficult because medical costs are skyrocketing for a number of reasons. New medications are expensive. You order one test for the patient and four for the lawyers. Doctors are so engrained in practicing that way. You could enact tort reform tomorrow* *and it will take five years to catch up. That adds grossly to the costs. A primary care shortage, you need them or you can hop from one specialist to another. You need someone to organize it and can see the whole forest not individual trees. How are you are going to save money by not paying doctors and hospitals. You are not going to get brighter people, you will get losers. Why am I going to come out with a debt of three quarters of million a year and be told that you will make $70,000 a year? No one but losers will do that. Bright people will do something else.*

- *Tort reform. You could save so much money. It is out of control. Talk to a doctor in the trenches.*

- *End of life care needs to be better addressed. The futility of care. The menu of offers to family members in ICU.*

- *It would be nice to be compensated better so that you don't have to see so many people. Independent.Running a company. Salaries and overhead. It would be great to be able to spend a half hour with every visit but you can't make it that way.*

- *End of life. We spent too much money on end of life care. Fighting DNRs within families. We need to stop doing everything for every patient. We need to make sure that we get advanced directives and ask again. They can become sicker. A large percentage of our medicine is spent on last six months or year of life. If you have an illness in the northwest, if you are not functional and can't work, can't communicate, they will not keep you going. You should not kill them. You do the basics, and you don't do such advanced care on somebody whose quality of life is so diminished. It's a massive amount of money. The hospitalists don't know them and they think that they don't care. There is a disconnect. The PCP is not in the hospital. They cannot survive to be there. Different doctors in several acute facilities and people are not prepared for this. They go back to the hospital. It's not the same person who they once had. They don't how to let go and be taught what is right about letting to. They need to understand what they are going to hold onto. So who is going to explain this to the families and patients? Look at all the money that has been spent to do that. That would be a tremendous reduction in health-care costs. How you limit care has to be done with committees and proper people, criteria and guidelines. In England you cannot be dialyzed after 75. In India, there is a corrupt system everything has to be cash. Kickbacks. They don't pay taxes. The Indian doctors can't live with that so they come here. You die in a public hospital. In England the social ystem is not bad, I was there, they had a good system. You got decent care the docs work 9-4:30 and made a decent salary. Then they go to private hospitals and practices. Let's go back 50 years came in before Medicare. There was a better balance.*

You are going to have some kind of socialization. Someone has to take care of the indigent. Some people have no money. Have to pay for someone to do it. There are different intelligences within the society and different expectations. The federal system is a duplication. Let them go anywhere. Trillions of dollars are wasted.

- *Obamacare. Most people don't understand the system, like my sister in Florida. She doesn't get it. Liberals don't understand the economics.*

- *I think that especially with the computer, they are trying to plug medicine. The EMR has a lot to do with it. They are trying to plug people into templates. You can't do that. Everyone has a different story, everyone is different. Similar but different.*

- *How to get everyone the care they need at an appropriate level. Our end of life care is a problem. A friend who does palliative care and helps the family have conversations about how they want the end of life to go. It's wasteful of resources and money and it's disrespectful.*

- *Lack of autonomy. The patients do not realize how much time it takes to fight with the insurance companies.*

- *Has to do with either the nature of underlying diseases and how to treat them and how are we going to afford to give all of the healthcare that people want.*

- *Insurance. It's ridiculous that I have to call them for permission. They refused to give permissions for a CT scan and finally she got it, and she had cancer. I could have gotten sued. I didn't. Everyone hates Obama but my sister is bankrupt and my son is 24 and is not working and they can get insurance.*

- *One is lack of access for a large segment of the population and the cost of increasing health care costs.*

- *Another unintended consequence. Should have just rolled everyone into Medicare and not hire all the new people and agencies. I don't know where it is going or where it will be in 10 years.*

- *The mismatch in goals.*

- *Healthcare policy.*

- *We have the evidence that we produce the best medicine in the world under a free system.*

- *One glove fits all cannot work. A poor person cannot have access to the president's doctor.*

- *Who is going to pay for it and how. People are so ignorant of what they need until they are in a health care crisis. Why they should be paying up front for insurance and why it costs so money. They don't understand how much nurses cost, heart monitors cost and everything that it costs to save their lives and how much the last two years cost when it will not bring them back to the life they knew. We have not educated our society about what it costs. People are dealing with loss and they don't understand reasonable outcomes and what it costs them and society about what it costs. People don't want to make these nasty decisions so that when illness happens there are unreasonable expectations. People expect doctors to fix everything at a low price. Health care has become a commodity like everything else and it is not working.*

- *We seek disease actively rather than focusing on wellness that will prevent disease most of the time.*

- *I don't think that we always understand what the goal is. To make people feel better? Improve quality of life? Make people live longer? Live forever? With one patient have I address what you came in for.*

- *It is so hard to get to the point of a doctor. We put off gratification that other people have. A shame to not earn money.*

- *How to provide high quality care. Educating people that not everybody lives forever. Patients have trouble understanding that public health affects them. Someone who has a real medical problem is not covered if people insist on what they don't need.*

- *The relationship between the insurance companies and the providers*

CHAPTER 5

THE HEALTHCARE CRISIS

What is the current state of healthcare?

* "Lots of physician burnout. The insurance companies seem to be the only ones making any money. The status of our current health is declining, not improving". Another doctor said, "It's a nightmare from every angle". Only a few tiny blips of positivity from the interviewees. Insurance companies are indeed making money. They trade on the stock exchanges and reward their shareholders while doctors are struggling to keep their doors open and make ends meet and patients are being denied healthcare. The salaries of their CEO's are "skyrocketing". Their "median pay... is higher than any other industry." This means "exceeding 10 million dollars." There are currently several lawsuits pending on the behalf of customers (patients) and providers accusing Blue Cross Blue Shield of operating as "an illegal cartel" and "price fixing."

• *Not great. When we compare out outcomes with other countries. C sections. Even with all the technology we have it's not great.*

• *Best healthcare system in the world but not for long.*

• *Fair*

• *Fragmented. Different rules about medicine for different people. You get what you pay for. If you have a good job and insurance, you are entitled to good care. With Medicare, if you are coerced into buying a managed care Medicare and cannot afford a supplement, you have fewer options with doctors and medicines. People don't know this and don't know what they are being sold.*

- *For me it means taking care of the patients. I don't look at the money aspect. I don't change my profession. I can't control how much money I make. It does not mean that my care of my patients will go down. But what I do see is doctors who are trying to make the same amount of money. They see more patients in less time which boils down to poor health care.*

- *Trying to provide good healthcare for a large number of people in an affordable way that still reimburses the providers a fair rate for their work. Hospitals and doctors. When I went into private practice in 1972, it was around the time the HMO's came in. They were horrible and then we came to a happy medium. Then the federal government came in with Obamacare and totally upset the apple cart. Now we are trying to figure out how to work with that. Meaningful Use, ICD-10 and Physician Quality Reporting System (PQRS) are here all at once and adopting EMRs and all of this is outside of patient care.*

- *It is a nightmare. From every angle.*

- *Troubled.*

- *It's such an overwhelming problem. Everyone wants a Mercedes. No one wants a Honda and everyone wants the government to give it free. People think that they are enti-tled to health care for free. Highly trained people taking care of them shouldn't cost them anything. Doctors got their fees cut so they turned us into businessmen. Labs tests. Trying to make up for the fact that fees are cut to a quarter than what they should be. Regulations and the people who practice good medicine get hurt. The people who can get around it still do it and still bleed the system. Targeting reforms at the doctors but not the insurance companies, or pharmaceuticals. Before HMOs people understood that if they want to the doctor they had to pay. So they made a decision to go or not. This vision of health care as an entitlement is different from 30 years ago.*

- *We are in deep doodoo. Seven hundred million dollars is taken after Medicare for Obamacare, which will hit the vulnerable. The hospitals are hit the worst. Unfunded liabilities and requirements. It's like any Ponzi scheme. The first guys do well.*

- *I have no idea. I live in my own bubble. I take care of my patients and I hope that I can continue to afford to do it. I hope that we focus on health and not sick people as a nation. Our biggest problem is obesity. Resources are not spread out properly. No one has really good national healthcare. We have good health care for those who can afford it. We fall short with the working poor.*

- *Losing money. Our marks on quality of care received is lower.*

- *We have always been in a healthcare crisis. The problems have always been there. We shine a light on them now and so it looks different. The presidents have always wanted to do healthcare reform. The doctor in me is not happy with some of the changes. The civilian in me believes that some of the changes are necessary. People who work without health insurance won't have it. It wouldn't pay me as much. But we see how it is. One nursing home has a sudden influx of people with no health insurance. They overlook their health their whole life.*

- *Everyone one is struggling. We are such little piece of a big puzzle.*

- *In transition. Obamacare is a start. At least make some progress.*

- *In this country. I think that we are not delivering as a good a product as we think that we are. There are some very discouraging statistics, like the infant mortality rate, that show us that access is a problem. It comes down to money and the insurance companies having too much power over the processes. Some of the problems reflect larger problems in society like poverty and education. My patients are insured and have jobs or are retired. Health care is not separate from other issues in society and when you have people who do not understand healthy choices and health it is often a result of no education. No access to education for the people who need it the most. We have a lot of work to do. Doctors and people going in to specialties, the cost associated with medical school is insane and choices after medical school are related to this. Or people don't want to go work in underserved areas when they have to pay their loans back. The education needs to be subsidized more.*

- *The computer makes it worse. It doesn't make it better. We don't use the computer in the room and so we run slowly and so the patients get pissed off. The insurance companies are in charge. They make everything so hard.*

- *A lot of things are good. We are getting patient centered and doing a better job reaching out to patients who are not here in the office. Encouraged re: Medicare chronic care management. That is good. Patient centered medical home. Some things are getting worse but many things are taking time and not improving things. The Accountable Care Organization (ACO) is doing good things. The data management is still in its infancy, i.e., pharmacy issues. This is among the stupid things.*

- *Not good*

- *Confusion*

- *Healthcare remains strong. But the business of healthcare is in turmoil. And if this crisis is not fixed, we will begin to see a worsening of the care provided. We are already seeing some degrading of care provided to patients across the country. Wait times are up. It is harder to schedule appointments. Patients are still flocking to the ER. Healthcare is sick. The management is in turmoil.*

- *It's a mess.*

- *As physicians we have made remarkable advances in our abilities to diagnose and treat human disease. With the financial crisis, and the current restrictions on practice caused by insurance companies, many physicians have changed the way they practice medicine.*

- *Abominable and it's immoral.*

- *Unstable*

- *Cost. It is rapidly becoming unaffordable. We are creating a class of uninsured. Millions of people are underinsured. They have insurance but it is not adequate to preventive basic care. We don't yet understand how to use technology and computers because we are spending incredible times documenting what we did and it is still hard to share with other providers. It is frustrating. Payment discriminating discrepancies that do not jibe with policy. So we have more of what we don't need and less of what we do need. We pay not enough psychiatrics general surgeons and family docs too much too radiologists too anesthesiologist and dermatologists. Also medical education is too damn expensive.*

- *Lots of physician burnout. The insurance companies seem to be the only ones making any money. The status of our current health is declining, not improving. We are so specialist driven. Lack of good primary care. Resources are being over utilized for some and underutilized for others. That is worse now than it used to be. Doctors are afraid of legal repercussions. So we have created a culture of just doing one more thing. We are afraid of sticking by our opinions. So we send people on to one more specialist and one more test to prove the one in a million chance. It makes me afraid to stick with my opinion as patients will just seek another opinion. It erodes the doctor-patient relationship. The stress of what's on us every day. The weight of carrying the burden of your health and the fear of repercussions is you think that we have made a mistake.*

- *Frightening. Abysmal. It will never be what it is. The pharmaceuticals are dying. They can't survive because the ACO's are demanding generics. It is so multi-tiered. The providers are wiped out and stressed. The insurance companies and pharmaceuticals are stressed. The hospital systems are stressed. They are buying up practices. I don't know what will happen. The last seven or eight years have been horrible. The last two years have been grotesque. The pre-authorizations are too time consuming.*

- *The healthcare costs are rising. The technology is increasing constantly and that is expensive. A significant chunk of the healthcare dollars go to administrative costs in the health care reform. I only see that increasing, i.e., EMR. A lot of information technology companies licking their chops with the push towards EMR in health care reform. We have gone overboard. Defensive medicine. Most of the docs, many I have spoke with, feel like they are sitting ducks in the legal system. Any potential outcome even if it has nothing to do with the care, just the disease process, may result in the doctor being sued. Defensive medicine and stress. There are bad docs and malpractice is out there and has to be looked at.*

Beyond that there is a lot of defensive medicine. One thing that has also changed over time is patient demands. Many people come in with a headache and expect and MRI or a CT scan or some significant testing. Most people don't need those tests. They also have potential side effects in addition to the significant costs. Radiation is a side effect. Try not to overuse. But it's tough. Requires a lot of discussion with the patients as they see it on House and in the media. Also a lot more false positives and incidental findings. Do a test for reason A, but an incidental finding shows up. May have no medical significance. Cannot be ignored and the doc has to follow up. We try and teach the residents and students — stepwise--do it when needed, not when not needed. It is all in the setting of defensive medicine. Health care reform has not looked at it enough yet. Defensive medicine and tort reform.

Another concern is increasing number of uninsured patients. A concern as a physician as well as a member of society. In my practice we do take care of uninsured and government insured patients. The big issue is that the numbers are increasing. Economy and job loss and the health care system hasn't figured out what it wants to be yet. Some initiatives have worked in small ways. More people are losing their insurance so we are still behind the eight ball. Even with insurance it has gotten more expensive and co-pays and deductibles are increased. We see more patients skipping their appointments and meds. I don't have the answer to it. It is a governmental/ societal issue has to be addressed. A consensus. Not necessarily socialize, but how will it progress, while at the same time, trying to control the costs. More healthcare isn't necessarily better, it's just more.

- *Abominable. I am in favor of a single payer Medicare system for everybody. I am also in favor of a fee schedule that doesn't put pressure on physicians to order more tests. Two reasons for it. It makes money. I love my doctors. They are under pressure every time I see them to order more tests. Sometimes it is being done for the bottom line rather than my needs. A lot of discussion in the papers about unnecessary testing.*

Misc

- *Who knows. It may be good. It may be terrible. I have no idea.*

- *Good. Patients are healthier than they were and living longer. People walking without canes and wheelchairs in their 90's.*

Q: How would you summarize the healthcare crisis?

* The same sorts of responses to this question as "What is the current state of healthcare". More comments here about the negative impact of insurance companies, entitlement, access, and lawsuits. Millions of Americans are uninsured. Obamacare is fraught with financial and access problems.

- *Not good.*

- *Insufficient providers of primary care in a world of increased specialization.*

- *It has to change. Nothing even makes sense right now. What Obama has done. New Jersey Governor Chris Christie screwed the state by expanding Medicaid. We can't even take it. If people don't get jobs they are one of the millions on the dole. We can't afford it. We are in dire straits financially. He should have stood with the other governors. These patients are so complicated and so sick. The clinics have closed.*

- *In total crisis.*

- *The bureaucracy is swallowing medicine. I would like everyone to have adequate health care insurance. There is a way to do it. But doctors are caught in the middle of a hijacking of medicine by people who don't understand medicine. We did not fight for our independent rights early enough, we are too busy and stressed out, and we let the currents take up and then complained about where we landed on the shore. The damage to the relationship. The insurance companies select ways and you cannot even pick your own doctor, they have to be on a list. This demystifies doctors and needs to be thought of by their patients to trust them. It's a complicated journey of cancer or birth, you have to surrender and trust and get in the ship with the doctor and go. Everything is breaking up the relationship and the patients are scared to death because they do not have their doctors. You have to have a certain mystique where people believed that we have an ability to heal and help. We have the experience. And I will know. It is frustrating and it disrupts the relationship. We are losing the idea that the doctors possess the skills and talent to heal. We need to get back to that or someday you will wake up sick and there is no one to take care of you or the doctor is too young or nervous and doesn't know you to care and to make a decision. Everything is eroding the trust and confidence in the doctors. We will lose the doctors and the whole system will fall apart. No one is doing it for the money anymore.*

- *Malpractice needs reform. This is where all the money goes. Can't take care of people when worried all the time about being sued. We need to subsidize medical education. Not coming out of education with $200,000 in debt. We need to start subsidizing education so that we attract good candidates.*

Good people are going into business. People are angry because they are paying and they don't know where the money is going. We lost house calls. Lost that piece of intimacy. If you are really sick and go to the hospital your doctor from the office will not be there. When the doctor was making enough money it made sense. We don't get paid enough now to work that hard and lose all of that quality of life. Our salaries are down. We gain quality of life. Patients pay less but they lose some continuity of care. The hospitalists are good and the patients will be well taken care of but it will not be my face that they see at the hospital. They will be well taken care of medically but they will lose that personal touch and we are not going to get it back.

- *Like many other current crises in this country and the world, a crisis of people being about to recognize and speak about limits and speak of them in an adult way without being demonized. Someone is always looking to take advantage of people who bring less than stellar news.*

- *People want free healthcare. The profit motive does not inure to the well being of the general population. If it is profit-driven then you are f'ed.*

- *The insurance companies have too much power. That needs to change.*

- *Confusion. So many rules and regulations it takes away time from the patients because I am watching to make sure that I am in compliance with all of this stuff.*

- *It is always in crisis. Medicine is in a perpetual state of flux. Those adept at dealing with change will survive and thrive. Those who are committed to traditional models will be dissatisfied. Nothing else.*

- *Like any business, there is only so efficient one can be until the services have to be compromised. We are at a point in healthcare where service is starting to be compromised. Unlike a dry cleaner or a plumber or an electrician, who may be able to cut corners, healthcare should never cut corners.*

- *In a nutshell: The destruction of the practice of medicine by third parties who profit from it. In my opinion to centrally control, to ask a bureaucrat what someone is feeling, it's impossible. But in government controlled medicine, that is necessary.*

- *I can't really summarize it easily. Probably it centers around quality of care and access to care. Most people put cost in there and that is part of the crisis. But you cannot control costs by getting people to do less. You have to cut out the middlemen.*

- *It has affected or limited and in some cases the tests we would like to order, the referrals we would like to recommend, or the treatments we would like to suggest. If I recommend an MRI and the insurance company refused to pay for it, this is a problem. Although CT scans can cause cancer scan in children, the insurance company will not pay for the MRI unless we do it first. How should I tell the child's mother? Send the child for PT so see if maybe they will get better? What if the best one is out of network and the parent chooses someone who is not very knowledgeable? It happens. This started changing five to ten years ago. This is wrong. We should be able to recommend the diagnostic tests, the therapeutic interventions, and the procedures that we think are necessary.*

- *Invented by the government. And it's showing that it's nefarious to be entrepreneurial in medicine and that government regulations would be here to protect everybody. However, government guidelines stress preventable care, whereas most studies today show that preventative medicine doesn't prevent disease.*

- *Because of the economics a lot of people have trouble paying. Costs go up. Keep trying to buy a cheaper and cheaper form, it limits your access to doctor or the doctor won't get paid and cannot afford to give the same amount to time. They can't afford to. If you run your office like an HMO mill with no choice, it will impact care and the doctor-patient relationship. PA's and office extenders, and you may never see a doctor or never hear about your case. It's dangerous. Many patients accept it. Many patients who downgrade understand. The malpractice situation has a lot to do with it. If you pay less and worry less about being sued over stupidity and wasting time, all costs could come down. Lawyers don't want to curb it. A huge problem. Also we give health care away for free to people who are not here legally. A family injured in Mexico, they would not let this family leave until they put $50,000 on their card. Other countries don't do that. They don't give it away for free. This is a huge drain. Giving more and more for free when you can't afford to is a problem.*

- *Insurance. People don't have it. Or they are tied to an employer. Having to ask for permission for meds or a test affects my day to day operations and the ability to refer a patient. There is a lack of information. People pay a lot of money and they think that should take care of it. They paid already.*

- *Obamacare meant well but it is not the problem. The insurance companies are the problem. How to make it fair to everyone? Patients do not understand.*

Q: IS THIS DIFFERENT THAN IT USED TO BE? IF SO, HOW?

* Yes, we have less access to quality healthcare. One doctor interviewee said, "We never had to worry about corners. It was always about the patients." Problems with insurance contribute to the denial of care. "Insurance companies weren't allowed to deem a recommended procedure as unnecessary, not indicated, and not reimbursable.", said one doctor interviewee.

- *More acutely aware of limits like economic and harder to avoid. The ability to deliver the increasing amount of healthcare that people demand. The resources are being stressed to the max and are going to shrink.*

- *It's worse. There used to be indemnity insurance. You could see who you wanted. Medicare is the Cadillac now.*

- *Oh yes. The denials of basic care. The number of mental patients incarcerated. The number of patients with Medicaid and these patients who have no one to take care of them. No thank you from any of the hospitals. No one has ever given us anything. No help from the insurance companies. We don't ask for money. We are clean. My patient with lupus. We are paying for it. Medicare rejected her and she is hungry.*

- *Obamacare right or wrong has brought this to the front. We talk about it.*

- *Medicaid and Medicare transformed stuff.*

- *The insurance companies did not have as much power dictating things to me in the past as they do now.*

- *Yes. We never had to worry about cutting corners. It was always about the patients, and everything else took care of itself. Now it is about the bottom line and whatever is left we put towards patient care. The best example is going to a doctor's office today and you will see that they are dirty with old chairs and they haven't been painted recently. Does anyone believe that the doctor wants an old office and a dirty waiting room? But you have to save it, whatever amount money, so they save it on the facilities and the cleaning of the facilities. You can tell how well a physician is doing based on the facilities.*

- *Insurance companies weren't allowed to deem a recommended procedure as unnecessary, not indicated, and not reimbursable.*

- *There is no shortage of people who want to inject themselves between the doctor and the patient and challenge our judgment. Who are these people? We backed out of one HMO 20 years ago. It's liberating not to answer to the third parties. I am immune to being so angry about the insurance companies.*

Misc

- *Better outcomes a long time ago. In the past we used to eat better and exercise better. We are good at treating advanced illness, not prevention.*

- *Yes.*

- *Who is saying it?*

- *No. it's just how the government wants us to think it is and that they can make it better.*

Q: WHEN DID YOU FIRST NOTICE?

* One interviewee said, "Slowly we have allowed this thing to creep up to the point to where we didn't even realize that we were losing control until it was too late. Gradually over a long period of time." Another one said, "Now it's every day."

- *A few years ago.*

- *Increasing in the past 20 years.*

- *HMO's, Managed care, PPO's.*

- *A few years ago. Now it's every day.*

- *1990s*

- *Medicare mandatory assignment. When the patient no longer paid. It was a third party system.*

- *Began to get obvious to me with the first reductions in Medicare in the late 1980s. HMOs in the 1990s. Aborted attempts to transfer healthcare in the 1990s, to the recent attempts – how will it work? Everyone seems to agree that there is not enough money for pay for an increasing rising volume of encounters and interventions and no one seems to know how to fix it.*

- *Late 70s and early 80s. I worked as a teacher and got fascinated with organizational change. Corporations noticed that their health care costs were out of control and this opened the door for managed care. They didn't know. They were promised equivalent care. They didn't know.*

- *Insurance has changed things in practice. You have to make decisions about which insurance to take based on what they pay. We couldn't afford it with some patients. The ACO negotiates rates which makes it a business which you have to have to keep your business going. It negotiates rates with the insurance companies. I am not that educated about it, but in countries with single payer there are problems with delays, with wait time and availability so that would have to be worked out, but we need better outcomes. It would not fix everything but it would help with access to quality health care and better outcomes. In Denmark, every mother who gives birth gets a box with supplies etc. to get them off to a good start and show them what they need. It can also be their first bassinette. A good message about how to take care of the baby. We need more public health minded solutions to problems. I wish we would do more.*

- *90s*

- *ACA and it is getting worse. The insurance companies are making money. Millions and billions of dollars are made by their CEO's. I just got paid last week for something I did six months ago.*

- *During the Clinton administration. Managed care. Managed care is another nail in the coffin of healthcare as we know it now. That is when physicians signed contracts with extremely low fees based on the promise of new patients, only the new patients never arrived and the fees became cemented in history.*

- *Slowly we have allowed this thing to creep up to the point to where we didn't even realize that we were losing control until it was too late. Gradually over a long period of time.*

- *There is no shortage of people who want to inject themselves between the doctor and the patient and challenge our judgment. Who are these people? We backed out of one HMO 20 years ago. It's liberating not to answer to the third parties. I am immune to being so angry about the insurance companies.*

Misc

• *I didn't notice anything.*

• *In the 40s and 50s with food and change in approach.*

• *Couldn't say.*

Q: WHAT IS WRONG WITH IT?

*Among other problems, "People are making decisions that they are not trained to make. They are not physicians."

• *Many things. Physicians are no longer able to advise what is best for them and do it and now must advise and then wait for an untrained person in front of a computer to approve or disapprove and then waste a huge amount of time fighting them. Patient doing really well on medication and the insurance company wants to switch them and then they do worse and then appeal to get them back on what was working before. Every day. I can't give you what is best for you sometimes. I can only give you what hopefully your insurance company will pay for.*

• *It will significantly decrease decision making between a doctor and his or her patients and will ultimately serve to restrict access via rationing. It affects the doctor-patient relationship will be based on protocols rather than handshakes. And this will ultimately disenfranchise the doctor-patient relationship as we know it. I have never practiced fee-for-service so can't tell you about the insurance.*

• *People are making decisions that they are not trained to make. They are not physicians.*

* One interviewee said, "There is no care of the patients, it's all about money."

• *Economic reward is driving it.*

• *People saw ways to make money in health care. It is a business.*

• *It's different than it used to be. In the 1908s my father was in full blown practice. The incentives changed. There is a financial incentive. We are not paid to think for office visits. The only thing that keeps us afloat is testing costs, equipment, and fancy things we do for people. But we want to cost contain. So they keep ratcheting us down, for example for office visits and professional fees for interpretation and thinking. Increases incentives to tests. There is no in between. Let's ratchet down testing by explaining and getting justification from insurance companies. This creates more positions in my department to make all of those phone calls and make it happen. It also makes patients unhappy. They have to wait days for the testing. Stressing about pre-authorizations. There is no care of the patients, it's all about money. There were abuses, from doctors, but this isn't working. It's bad.*

Q: How and why did this happen?

* Greed.

• *A few doctors and patients who ruined it for many. A few patients who ruined it for everyone. That is always the way.*

• *The HMOs taught people to be entitled and gave us less fees.*

• *The insurance companies saw this as a way of increasing their profits.*

• *Because doctors signed contracts before they read it.*

- Insurance greed. Need to talk the profit margins out of the insurance business. There is no reason for the CEO of one to get $8 million but you have to switch a patient to a different medicine because it will save a few dollars.

- Doctor abuse. Patients' expectations. I need expensive testing to be well, or my doctor is no good. Loss of confidence and doctor-patient relationship. The insurance companies make it too hard to get testing. Too much pre-authorization. The primary physicians cannot handle it so they send to the specialists even when I might not have anything to add clinically.

- The insurance companies control everything.

Q: How does this affect you as a doctor?

* It negatively affects care and the insurance companies play a role.

- A lot. Constantly trying to reverse damage that has already been done.

- Takes away money and time. There are CEOs, stock holders, boards of directors. Less time with patients. Less access to some of the things that they need. You have to fight hard and can get it. But you have to do a jig and a dance.

- When I see doctors recommending tests I would not do or do not understand end of life care. Why? Money.

- It enables them and makes them weak but it also keeps out people who really need access.

- It does not permit me to provide the best possible care for the patients. The insurance company dictates what I can and cannot prescribe.

- *It affects me because I manage the practice. The physicians who care for our patients are unaffected. In our practice we still practice medicine the old fashioned way. It is a struggle to provide that luxury to our physicians but it is something that I want to do as long as I possibly can.*

- *Obviously, if I am going to get a government paid position, all the competition factor is eliminated.*

- *This completely changes the role we play as physicians The insurance companies are taking the ability to practice medicine the way we want to away from us.*

- *It makes me less efficient, distracted, frustrated. The ratio of what I like and don't like is skewed.*

- *I sold the practice.*

Q: HOW DOES IT AFFECT THE PATIENTS?

* "The patients will be seen just like numbers or statistics," said one interviewee. It affects "accessibility and care."

- *It will affect them. Medicare is best. For others – big problem. More and more doctors will drop out of insurance. People called us and cursed. I knew them for 20 or 25 years and people don't appreciate it.*

- *Need for help.*

- *Too much suffering.*

- *They feel alienated, hopeless, and angry and depressed.*

- *Patients from before who say they couldn't afford our new practice and they resent it.*

- *Accessibility and care.*

- *They get inferior care.*

- *Our patients are spoiled. They don't feel the pain of healthcare. Patients don't have money; we help them. If they have lost their insurance, we help them. The only visible sign of the changing of healthcare may be that the waits are longer than I would like them to be but I expect every patient to be seen immediately either with an appointment or when they walk in, so maybe it is me that's unreasonable.*

• *The patients will be seen just like numbers or statistics.*

• *Delays in diagnosis. Delays in treatment. And in some cases I had to cancel surgery because of insurance reasons.*

• *They don't get adequate care sometimes. The ladies spend time on the phone. Hospitals buying up practices is going to ruin medicine. They micromanage practice and they don't know what to do. They are so demanding. They are ruining my practice.*

Q: How does it affect the doctor-patient relationship?

* It "puts stress on it" and "almost destroys it."

• *Influenced by less time to interact with the patients.*

• *Puts stress on it. But most patients realize that if you are the type of doctor who goes after what you need, less stress. They worry about the doctor who won't do the test or get the right meds. They worry about that. If you do the exceptions and paperwork, they know you are trying.*

• *The government and insurance are coming between the relationship. It is a doctor-payer relationship. They are trying to save money but are being paid huge amounts of money. If the government would work on that and limit that stuff more. The insurance intervention is becoming more and more difficult. You used to be able to write for any drug you wanted. Then if a non-preferred drug would cost the patient more this year we are not going to pay for it. You can fill out an authorization but we are not going to pay it. So you are paying full freight. Some insurance companies are telling me which generic to cover. A lot of people work for big companies and they have not yet felt the pinch of Obamacare. Talk to people with left leaning and they don't get it.*

- *The sense of entitlement and the sense that I should be able to fix everything that is wrong with them and they have no responsibility and that I should be their servant.*

- *Sometimes they think that they can't trust me so they never open up.*

- *It probably affects me less because I don't let it enter the discussion. I examine them blind to their carrier. They all get the same level of care. The difference is in the discretionary things where people have to be able to afford to purchase it, or if they can't be referred to certain people because there are not in their plans.*

- *It affects the relationship. As much as you try, you have to spend less time with the patients. Have to squeeze more people in. When you do have too many people you are seeing you cannot keep up with them all.*

- *Yes. Financial and insurance end. Some plans require fights to get tests and specialists. This all drives a wedge into me and my patient and I resent it.*

- *They understand that I want to prescribe drug A but I cannot do it. They do not take it as a personal thing on me.*

- *It screws it all up. I try to be nice, but the poor people…*

- *Managed care was the first wedge between the doctor and the patient. This was brought about by the fact that some doctors participated and some did not. If your physician participated, your patient had a small co-pay and it became evident that a small co-pay was more important than a long-term established doctor- patient relationship became obvious immediately. The relationship has blown up in the face of those who wanted it destroyed. It took the leverage away from physicians. The problem is that it also increased health care costs. As I said earlier, when you don't have a doctor-patient relationship you don't have compliance and then costs go up. They go up because patients who are not compliant have worse outcomes, and also when the doctor and the patient do not have relationship, the physician is more likely to over test to reduce the chance of malpractice. Most malpractice is a result of a poor relationship with the doctor and the patient.*

• *Almost destroys it.*

• *Irreversible. Now almost anything we do we have to really think about the cost-benefit ratio to the patients.Will the insurance company pay? If not, can the patient afford it? Will the patient be physically harmed if they don't get it? How can I help this patient?*

• *Patients get annoyed when their doctors cannot get testing done. They think that it is stemming from us. They don't see it as a systemic problem.*

• *It makes it more difficult to make them happy.*

• *Affected by advertising. Drug advertising on the TV and radio pushes patients to ask for treatments that may or may not be safe, that need to be individualized. Plus the biggest problem with the advertising is that they are full of lies. So many things are said in these commercials.*

Q: Has the insurance situation changed being a doctor? If so, how?

* Particularly disturbing quotes from two interviewees: "The insurance companies do not want patients to live. They make more money if the patients die." And, "Totally. I don't have patients, I have contracts with the insurance companies and so do the patients and I am the middle man."

• *Since I finished residency we have had HMOs. It used to be fee for service.*

• *With finances.*

• *I make occasional compromises on formularies.*

• *I am sick of the paperwork.*

• *Insurance pays more sometimes and sometimes less. Sometimes people would come in if they didn't have to pay. Sometimes we would tell them to come back if we knew that it would cost nothing.*

• *Yes. It used to be in the days of yore you provide the services you thought were appropriate. People were happy and there was no restraint. Now there are restraints via insurance companies willing to pay what they are entitled to and what we can offer.*

• *Some people say that they beginning of Medicare was the beginning of the problem. But no one can pay for medical care. If you have a headache, do you need a CT scan? No. The insurance company will pay for it and your doctor wants to get paid. Ok if it is a harmless test, but add it all up, but you have to scrimp somewhere else. It's America, you can have whatever you want. Money in the last months of life, the family members are unrealistic. Snippets of a bigger issue. In some countries people just don't get things, like dialysis. We need to cut out the middlemen, the insurance companies and put those billions back into the system. Half of the staff does case management and discharge planning and it doesn't help the patients. The nurses are charting, not taking care of the patients.*

- *The pot is not infinitely deep but you have to be efficient, and the way that costs are being constrained is not efficient and it gets in the way of my relationship with the patients.*

- *Yes. The insurance companies have too much power to dictate what I can and cannot do. This is disproportionate to their mandate. Their job is to provide the funds. They have too much power. They use this mandate, their interest is profits and any way they can increase it they can do it. Many physicians who are good people and do a good job have been penalized. Don't paint everyone with the same brush.*

- *Yes. The reason it has is because it is a struggle. The general public believes that as a physician you can negotiate with an insurance company. The general public doesn't read EOBs. The general public doesn't realize that what you charge is not what you collect. Imagine going to your lawyer, having him charge you a thousand dollars so for a service and you telling him you are only going to pay $300 and he had to accept the fee. That is what it is like dealing with insurance payers. In the old days when insurance companies paid reasonable fees, Medicare was the outlier for being the lowest fee schedule. Physicians accepted this fee schedule as it was their duty and because the other payers helped to even out the score. Over time the tables have turned and now Medicare, which still remains a low fee schedule, is now one of the best. And so doctors' ability to provide charity to provide charity care has been reduced.*

- *Totally. I don't have patients, I have contracts the insurance companies and so do the patients and I am the middle man.*

- *In the last five to 10 years more and more patients are sent out of state. They will find someone in network. Referred to a physician who is not a specialist in that area. First one was sent to two or three doctors for a problem because the insurance company doesn't want to pay. Finally to me. The surgery went fine.*

- *The insurance companies do not want patients to live. They make more money if the patients die.*

- *My major issue is pre-authorization is strangling me and my colleagues.*

- *Before insurance there was more accountability. The patient paid and saw what I did. It allowed us to really function as professionals and allowed a marketplace. We couldn't afford technology and if you got sick you were screwed. So we created health insurance, which we needed, but it took away accountability between doctor and patient. Swinging back to more accountability but it still has to be affordable so still need third party payment.*

- *I am sure that it has changed since I retired in terms of preapproval. I don't like the fact that some nonmedical person is asked to make the approval of a treatment or procedure before it is done*

Misc
- *Not really. I combined all of these.*

Q: WHY ARE THE PATIENTS SO RELUCTANT TO UNDERSTAND THE PROBLEM?

* "Unrealistic expectations" and "Entitlement."

- *People have this idea that more technology is better. If you don't order a lot of test of heroic measures are not done think that you are not a good doctor. Unrealistic expectations. Medicare is done in the last part of life and means procedures and tests that should not be done. Babies at 23 weeks with procedures that should not be done.*

- *Entitlement.*

- *They have been infantilized and taught that they shouldn't have to pay. Yet for cigarettes, the plumber, smart phone, car mechanic, they pay. Their health is the most important. And they don't expect the plumber to file with health insurance. You pay your bill. They present it to you and you pay. People are incensed at the end of a visit when they are presented with a bill. Do a surgery, save a kid's life. They take the money from the insurance company and keep it. Sometimes I do things for free, but I don't keep the check from the insurance company.*

- *They can't get what they want when they want it.*

- *The entire society. The society has changed. When I grew up you wanted to help everyone and cared. The society has turned to me. Entitlement. You don't matter. You should contribute to my entitlement.*

- *Every patient wants the best testing and care but they do not want to pay. They do not want to pay a nickel.*

- *A belief, facilitated by the administration over the last few years, that everything should be for free.*

- *I don't know. Many of them experience frustration who like to have their limits in their favor on a daily basis.*

* They blame the doctors.

• *They blame us all the time when it's the insurance. I see it all the time. I don't blame them. Why should they understand it? They have their own lives to worry about.*

• *Nobody is giving them the information. They hear what the media says and the media is very left-leaning and it is not affecting their pocketbooks yet. Some young kids are getting insurance through Obamacare and the older people are going to HMOs and then they come back. They save money but they are being told what they can and cannot do. A lot of patients think that the doctors are doing this. The doctors are money grubbing and they don't care, it could all be fixed if the doctors weren't millionaires. It is frustrating. The other thing that frustrates me is about income inequality; why don't we fix the job equality situation? I am cynical and we are approaching a socialist society where big government is taking care of everything and you can't get ahead. This country was made great by people who worked hard.*

• *The reason is because the problem is complicated and it is not their fault. They just want the care and people have a hard time being upset for a group that they feel are receiving what they perceive as fair compensation for their services.*

* Some of them understand, but it is complicated.

• *The economy sucks and people are having a hard time.*

• *Most haven't been affected by these problems until they get sick.*

• *I think that they understand. They resent their insurance and what they pay and don't pay and are allowed to do it.*

• *They are more understanding now that it's in the paper.*

• *They want to believe.*

- *I don't know if they are reluctant. Nature abhors a vacuum. A lack of understanding and rushes of voices come in to fill the void.*

- *Because it is too complicated.*

- *I think a lot of them do understand it. I hear patients complaining now about insurance.*

- *People are so overwhelmed. Information overload and financial stress. People feel since they can't change the system, why bother trying?*

- *They don't get it.*

- *They pay premiums and they think that's it. Medicine has become digitized and their own personal doctor. They are using medicine as a commodity like anything else. It is not the art of the profession, and the judgment and training are not reflected in a blog. Wonderful to become increasingly informed but not informed about things they know nothing about.*

- *It's really not ignorance to understand something that they don't think that exists. Someone is already paying for it and they don't care who is paying.*

Q: WHY ARE THEY SO ANGRY ABOUT IT?

* They feel powerless and helpless.

- *But they feel powerless to change it. It's easy to turn about and blame the physician, someone who you know and trust. Some people will be angry at me that they have to pay a co-pay. Mad that they have to pay a deductible. Hire a social worker to help people to talk to their insurance company. The insurance companies make them feel helpless and give up.*

- *They complain about their insurance and what it will let them do. My doctor is in the plan, this drug was working and I can't take it; I do not hear about it directed at me. It is directed at insurance companies and employers, who opt for some low cost insurance plan.*
- *They feel helpless.*
- *They feel as if they have lost choice.*

* Entitlement
- *They think that Medicaid patients get everything and everyone else gets nothing.*
- *They have been taught that they do not have to pay.*
- *It depends. Some people want everything for free. The ones who are the most angry take their patient relationship rights to the extreme.*

* "They don't understand."
- *They aren't. They don't understand.*
- *They think that it is us, the doctors, causing the problems. They are starting to understand that it is the insurance companies, not our inability to get them what they need.*
- *When someone doesn't pay for it they get angry. The problem will occur when their access is denied and they realize that it is not access denied, it's payment denied. As people become less healthy and morbid in some way, the anger may occur because of restriction to access, which is inevitable. Those societies we have been compared to all restrict access.*
- *It's too obtuse. They don't understand why hospitals have thousands of dollars of spiraling cost. It's a messed up reimbursement system and doctors and patients and get*

caught between it. I get frustrated when caught between the patient and insurance and patients do not understand that it is often the employer who bought the plan.

Misc

• *I don't know.*

Q: What are some solutions to the healthcare crisis? What has to change? How can this happen?

* "We have to reduce costs of care and I mean administrative costs of care. Transition those resources to patient care," said one doctor interviewee. Another said, "Go back to the old fashioned doctor. Like the 70s and 80s, sit down and talk to patients. Now you are just shuffling patients in and out. No passion. It's dull. They have to see a certain number of patients to cover overhead. Reimbursements are down and patients are demanding."

*Insurance and malpractice reform

• *Nobody is willing to make serious decisions. If we have national health insurance decisions have to be made about what the government will not pay for IVF, last six months of life, 23-weekers, termination of pregnancies, circumcisions. Have to make these decisions, no discussions. In other countries, someone has to decide who will pay for it. Need a limit. Need to realize what is really going on. I think there are some areas of the country that are overloaded with certain types of physicians and some where we do not have enough. Have to make decisions about where MDs will practice.*

• *By our insurance style and dominance of the insurance in control of the system.*

- *A simplified one payer system would be better but no one solution. It's too complicated and convoluted.*

- *Leave it alone. Or single payer system. Can buy a supplement. Too much free stuff in this country. No skin in the game.*

- *Pay for what we do and take us out of business ie diagnostics labs. But double our fees that we get paid. Something has to be done with pharmaceutical companies from making drugs that we don't need and not advertise to create need. We need innovation. It needs to change life with reward and financial reward for hard work but on a limited scale. Other incentives to get pharma to work on medicines to change people's lives. No repackaging of off-patent drugs. Having insurance be for profit is a problem. I do think that government should have a stronger role in healthcare. HIPPA is a piece of sh.t. However, I can order 10 million extra tests and line my pockets and its okay. Medicine has been taken out of the hands of the people who provide good care. There are some bad doctors but most of us are ethical and we have to wade through the morass.*

- *Put tort reform on the agenda and the insane litigation, it is a cost we are all bearing. It has to be tort reform, it costs nothing to sue us over nothing and then we are supposed to settle. People have to take some responsibility of costs. If everyone had to pay it they would be less flippant about wanting an MRI because they knew costs. Put some of the financial benefit on the patients. They have to be a player and will pick, for example, generic medications.*

- *Having an intelligent bipartisan discussion as to how third party payment for health care is going to be shaped and limited and what options private people have. Can they purchase extra service other than what is offered by a bureaucratic body?*

- *I don't know the answer. Insurance companies. The major providers who want to drive data streams. No one expects car insurance to pay for oil changes. But everyone expects health insurance to pay for everything. Astounding technology but we have lost the human touch. The public will always over consume what is for free.*

- *Just pay for it. It would be easier. (insurance)*

- *Single payer system. Eliminate the insurance company profits, administrative costs and bureaucracy. Medicare for all. For the politicians not to be taking campaign contributions from the insurance industry.*

- *The system is so screwed up. How do you unscrew it? Insurance companies are driven by money. Politicians. They don't care. You need to unwind it and redo it. A lot of things in the ACA that were not in the states were in New Jersey. No pre-existing conditions and you can move to other companies. How is the best way to get the uninsured insured? I would have put them all under Medicare. It works.*

- *We have to reduce costs of care and I mean administrative costs of care. Transition those resources to patient care. There has to be a fair playing field with regards to fee schedules. Hospitals should not be paid more for services in their hospital or one of their clinics than is performed in a physicians' office. We have to continue to find processes and protocols that provide good outcomes. But we also can't lose sight of the fact that health care is as much an art as it is a science.*

- *Malpractice reform. Free market in medicine as much as possible. Opening the barriers to trans-state insurance business which will stimulate a price reduction.*

- *I don't have the answer. My theory and most of my doctor colleagues do not agree. I think you need a single payer system. The problem is the same as monarchy. Every dictator will not be benign.*

- *We want everything done right away and this will not happen with socialized medicine.*

- *Don't know. I can list for you what is wrong with Europe, Israel and Canada.*

- *There should be a conscious and fair redistribution of wealth, but not the way some people talk about it. It's not the 99 percent. The ultra ultra rich. There are no ultra rich physicians. CEOs make millions. Some pediatricians make less than an office manager. The insurance companies have sold doctors as greedy and rich. This is not the case. A few bad apples, i.e. sports. The World Series a baseball game. Let's talk about where some of the real problems are.*

- *It is not an easy answer. But what is going on now isn't working. The number one problem is the malpractice crisis. That has to go. Once the lawyers are out of that, it will be easier.*

- *I don't have the mechanism but it has to be not capitated. It can't be a free for all either. This precertification by controlling certain entry points isn't working. Remunerate clinical decision making better. Pay people to think about their patients not see so many patients and have no time to think about them. Take away some of the administrative crap like having to understand 80 insurance companies and stop shutting down offices that can't meet the expectation. Judge based on other than codes and paperwork. The ratios are a distortion. We have to hire people to prevent losing money. Lower reimbursements by demanding so much administrative work that we can't comply.*

- *Would really be a system where preventative care is covered on a sliding scale basis including a deductible where patients would have skin in the game where the insurance companies or the government would step in after a set sliding fee scale. When people have skin in the game they don't abuse the system. The average American does not have risk in the payment game and that's what the problem is. For my daughter's acne medicine, I called other pharmacists and had skin in the game and called around I saved myself $300 a month. $5 ear symptoms – someone came in to see my wife before they went on a trip to get their child's ears checked. They had no symptoms, but it only cost $5, so they did it. People are going to get what they wanted. They wanted shift workers and that's what they will get.*

- *I don't know. Everybody has to give a little. I am not in this business to know the good old days. For me it has always been uphill.*

- *Go back 20 years. It's too late. We are in a downward spiral to deterioration and demise. The environment in the hospital. We all used to know each other like a family trying to provide care. Now everything is so fragmented, antagonistic, and layered. Multi-tiered non- communicating layers. I am very sad to see it happen. We are much better at providing remedies. But not with personal care. Some people see 50 patients a day. How do they do that? That will never provide decent care.*

- *Direct pay, high deductible insurance and real charity. We feel special here as opposed to the hospital. Doctors will be heroes again for donating their time to justify the tremendous sacrificed time, education, and lost income.*

- *A single payer Medicare like system for everybody.*

* Go back to the future and provide better health care.

• *Go back to the old fashioned doctor. Like the 70s and 80s sit down and talk to patients. Now you are just shuffling patients in and out. No passion. It's dull. They have to see a certain number of patients to cover overhead. Reimbursements are down and patients are demanding. It is a lot more difficult to pleased patients and to try to keep everything calm. When they leave this door you don't know what will happen. You will hear about it at some time or other. It can shake me up. Things still stick with me from nine years ago.*

• *I can't imagine that. We are no longer innocent. We are tainted like so many other parts of our society. I worry about me as an older person. Who will take care of me and care about me?*

• *Having doctors that are actually dealing with it. Having them more involved in the decisions being made to improve it.*

• *The relationship we have with our patients will diminish. Go into bigger practices and we are less in tune to what patients need as opposed to just on a physical level. Hoping not to lose it. But we will.*

Misc

• *We are communists.*

Q: WOULD YOU SHARE SOME OF YOUR FEELINGS ABOUT IT ALL?

• *I am skipping to insurance. I have problems with high deductible plans including Obamacare. You penalize somebody. You make them pay for insurance. The insurance will cost them $2,500 to $5,000 a year and now you are going to make them have a $2,500 deductible. Now these people outside of one free physical a year do not have* *insurance. I have a policy in my office if one of my patients does not have insurance we charge $50 for a visit. We have a deal with a lab to discount their lab prices. And I have a wide array of generic medications that I can pick. Patients with diabetes and no insurance that see me 4 times a year I can see them for $1,000 year. That same person now went from $9,000 to $5,000 for insurance and now my visits are going to be $75-100 and I can't discount it because the patient has insurance. A person just got mandatory government insurance and their costs went up. $5,000 per year. And they are supposed to say thank you.*

I am sick of it. People with regular insurance. Even the Obamacare insurance is high deductibles. So I am fielding phone calls for people debating the bill because they want me to put it as an annual physical but you get only one annual physical. So now they don't want to come in. So I am wasting my time calling people. Another level of interference between me and the patient. It's another wall that gets put up. Patient comes in with pain and they are hesitant to get the testing done. They may not get the test due to financial reasons. I have to worry about it because of health and legal. If this person has a ruptured appendix and they didn't go because of money the lawsuit won't say that. Or no routine colonoscopy for the same reasons, somehow it's my fault. I am trying to get them to do it and they don't want to do it. It can become antagonistic. I have an insurance company rating me on my percentage of people getting colonoscopy or pneumonia shots, all good things to get. It's like I am pestering them and they don't want to do it and they get mad.

- *I would end by saying quality of care should never be sacrificed and I believe that the key to quality care is the*

*doctor-patient relationship. And the powers that be
intentionally put a wedge between physicians and patients.
Without patients advocating for physicians, no one listens.
In most my colleagues I see the kind of care that they are
forced to provide. Everyone knew that more patients would
be covered under the ACA but that the quality of care would
suffer. There has to be a way to improve access and increase
quality. I am afraid that the path we are currently on does
the opposite.*

*And it used to be that there were lots of doctors in country
clubs. They can't afford it now. The same thing with nice
cars. There was a social pact in place: we provided care and
we had a comfortable life. That pact was broken. The deal
was broken. So now there is a new generation with a new
attitude: We will provide care when we want to provide care,
9-5 and no weekends.*

- *That's all in relation to your questions. One thing that I
look forward to in medicine are more multi-specialty groups
under the same roof. I see primary care. I used to go with
experience. I now go with youth. The ones who were experience
all retired when I retire. Now I have a 30-year-old who will
be around when I am not. My nephrologist is a 35-year-old
woman. My cardiologist is a middle aged man whose children
were patients of mine. One thing that is good about modern
medicine is communication. It is fantastic. I go for an X-ray
and my doctor can pull it up on a computer so that we can
look at it together. I had a surgical problem about two years
ago. My doctor didn't think he could do it and he referred
me to another vascular surgeon elsewhere. That kind of
behavior is what I expect for anyone. He was good but knew
his own limitations. He knew that this other guy could do it
better. I did it and I am doing very well.*

Something needs to be done about the malpractice situation. A special court system made up of judges made up of consultants who are specially trained should handle the problem.

I did enjoy it. Medicine.

What I hear about medical education these days. It's different. More technology is involved. When I was trained we listened to patients' hearts. The students now listen to a dummy's heart. In some medical schools they don't dissect cadavers. They do it on a computer. The impact of technology is mixed.

Another solution to the problems in this country would be if we had more doctors. If the medical schools could increase their enrollment.

Another thing that is happening is the development of subspecialties. There are so many of them, i.e. an orthopedic surgeon who does only hands or elbows. Carving up medicine into too many subspecialties.

And I do not like the government getting involved in medical issues like contraception and abortion.

Q: What has been lost?

* Patient care and the doctor-patient relationship, so important to care, compliance and also to cost containment, has been lost. This was explained clearly by the doctor interviewees in the beginning of this book.

• *Patient care. Lots of tests is not patient care. Drawing a lot of labs, that's not patient care.*

• *Individuality and the rare exception of the close relationship with the patient.*

- *Freedom.*

- *It takes a lot of the fun out of being a doctor and takes a lot of the relationship away.*

- *The attention to the patient.*

- *Our respect for physicians. For health. Understanding that health is not a given right. It is something that you work for and you have to be an active participate in it. Doctors are human and we make mistakes.*

- *We have lost some spontaneity. Some informality. Intimacy. Everything is very stylized. We will never get that back. The world has changed. The rules will always be hovering in front of us in a way that they did not in the past. May have an upside. Doctors should never have unlimited latitude to do with patients. Still needs to be a break in unnecessary suffering caused by the relentless attempt to milk a few more moments of life spending hundreds of thousands of dollars in the process.*

*Ah, those insurance companies and malpractice problems again.

- *My summary is back to basics. I think that the insurance companies are the problem. All of the third party payers have caused the price problem. No one can afford $2,000 for an MRI. Prices would come down. A complete disconnect between the cost of health care and the patient. The costs are uncontrollable. There needs to be tort reform. Defensive medicine. The doctors are just doing it to cover themselves. If you don't do it and get sued, it's an issue. I would make people who lose these cases pay the doctors.*

- *The litigation is horrible, the lack of autonomy. The amount of time for preapproval fighting with insurances it is time taken away from being with patients. The monetary is not a big worry list at the moment for me. We would all like to make more money, but...*

- *I don't know if there was a "good old days." There have always been problems with inequality and lack of access. But we have to start addressing these issues if we care about peoples' lives.*

- *In 1965 Medicare and Medicaid started the problems. A huge infusion of money and everyone wanted some.*

Misc

- *Life is dynamic. If something goes wrong, we are driven to change it. Nothing is wrong. We are just two people sitting in a room and there are 2 billion people in the world and we are comfy in our own little world.*

Q: CAN WE GET IT BACK? HOW?

* Not a lot of optimism here.

- *I don't think so.*

- *That is a difficult question. It's a matter of time to see how things roll out in the future.*

- *You cannot get anything today because of the political system. Both sides probably have good intentions. But they will not compromise.*

- *I don't know. I would still do it all over again. I would still go into the profession again. Probably. Everything cycles around and back. People won't like getting lost in the corporate structures.*

- *I have no idea. I doubt it. Healthcare is expensive and people expect perfect outcomes and that is impossible.*

- *With a miracle.*

- *I don't know. If so it will be past my time. It will be a generational shift.*

- *People need to stand up for their rights. Go to the Department of Banking and Insurance (DOBI). Let insurance companies know that this is not fair and unacceptable. When people sign on for an insurance policy, the insurance companies purposefully do not represent their actions and what they will and not cover in a way that is possible to understand. I had a guy come in and talk about 401 k's and I couldn't understand it.*

- *I don't know. We need leadership that understands the medical profession and is willing to stand up and say so. As long as people look at medicine as patsies and to be taken advantage of it won't happen.*

- *Duty hour restrictions are just for trainees so there is more stress on the supervising MDs. There is no give in the system. We work long hours and are on call. Stressful. The other concern as a program director will the patients be ready when they get out there. They are restricted and do more shift work – a more difficult transition to the practice paradigm.*

Mental health — mention that we are seeing more mental health issues in our patients. Is it because we recognize it? I don't think so. There are more mental health issues. The stress of society and expectations of society. Our connectedness. Technology stresses us out. Always connected to the internet or the mobile device and the information overload. Thus the need for more quality mental health providers and accessible especially uninsured or insured worse, underinsured. None of it is covered. Or by someone they can see within a 50-mile radius or has the expertise.

Insurance? The insurance companies have helped to create an increasingly complex bureaucracy that becomes more intimidating to navigate and understand for providers and patients. Stresses both out. I have seen people patients just give up. Have to keep working with the complexities and encourage patients and colleagues.

Misc

I want to be reasonable and balanced here.

SUMMARY AND IMPLICATIONS

* I learned that the healthcare crisis is worse than I ever imagined. For many, the insurance companies are dictating rationed, inadequate and insufficient health care. This leaves the fine men and women doctors who I interviewed, as well as their colleagues, in a totally untenable situation. I cannot say enough to adequately do this point justice. I do believe that the interviews in this book expose an intimate portrait of the gravity and urgency of our healthcare crisis.

To me, what is both startling and disturbing is the contrast seen when looking at the reasons doctors go into and continue to find value and merit in practicing medicine and the way they are treated by all the players in the healthcare system. Their explanations of how and why they care are incredibly moving. Their willingness to answer what most of them view as a calling, which they expected to be demanding, is profound. The interviewees make these points clearly in a number of different ways. Chapter 2 asks direct questions about why the interviewees became doctors, and the interviewees make the same point over and over all throughout the interviews. Many of the most disturbing answers are in Chapter 4 and 5.

Being a doctor is demanding clinically. This is coupled with the inability to practice medicine in a way that is both consistent with how they have been trained and what their clinical judgment tells them is the best care. The responsibility of the insurance companies in creating and maintaining the healthcare crisis comes through loudly and clearly.

- *So many people overseeing you. People don't respect us. What if every single decision has to be justified to a pre-law student with one political science course – to my sister in law – a judge. I spend my day talking to idiots with a book of algorithms. If you say the wrong word they deny the treatment.*

- *Gradually, as the insurance companies took over, they squeezed the doctors. Then came managed care and they managed the doctor. And the doctors were seduced into them. Now we are being seduced into being employees. Now you can no longer advocate for patients or you lose your job.*

- *I expected to be around tough and hard cases. I expected it to be hard. I did not expect to have to think if the insurance company will not pay for it.*

- *Healthcare should never cut corners.*

- *How can a procedure recommended by a doctor be deemed medically unnecessary? It should not even exist.*

- *People are making decisions that they are not trained to make, as they are not physicians.*

- *The insurance companies do not want patients to live. They make more money if the patients die.*

- *You are told by others with no experience with medicine how to practice and how to treat. You cannot sometimes give the best treatment to a patient because of bureaucrats who want to tell you to give second best or less best treatments."*
- *They think that it is us, the doctors, causing the problems. They are starting to understand that it is the insurance companies not our inability to get them what they need.*

- *It does not permit me to provide the best possible care for the patients. The insurance company dictates what I can and cannot prescribe.*

* What an absurd situation. Doctors are prevented from practicing properly. In training it is by duty hours and in practice it is by the insurance companies. But they are still held accountable for decisions that are not theirs.

* The most important part of medicine to these interviewees, the doctor/patient relationship, is being destroyed. This comes through in the interviews when asked about it directly and as part of other questions.

- *There is no care of the patients; it's all about money.*

- *I don't have patients, I have contracts with the insurance companies and so do the patients and I am the middle man.*

- *That is the problem now. The relationship has been chipped away. They try and take it away. And some doctors now are blind like robots. It's easier. If you invest in them, they switch anyway. Everyone is against you. So you pull back and withdraw. You do not want to be a target and getting attacked. IT HURTS when you are being attacked. Meanwhile when you get sick, who is taking care of you? Who calls your insurance to advocate for you? The patients are so entitled. They expect you to do it. They yell if it's not fast enough. The patient has a lot to do with the relationship and they are like spoiled brats. They go online and go to the insurance companies. They are taking everything even self esteem away from the doctor.*

- *I don't see the accountability and people saying 'I have to eat better, stop smoking and exercise'. The onus is on us*

*to do everything. There is pressure on us to do things that
we cannot do. How can we make them do things? No
accountability. If I didn't document well and something
happens, it could be a real problem. Sometimes you are in
a rush on the phone, in the hospital and shopping and tell
them what to do and you can't document everything.
So busy. If there is a bad outcome. No matter how
unaccountable the patient is for their own health they will
blame the physicians 9 out of ten times.*

- *The patients will be seen just like numbers or statistics.
The dedication of these doctors is not adequately rewarded,
financially or otherwise.*

- *This society accepts no mistakes. And in any job that
people perform – in any job it will never be 100% perfect.
The public needs to understand that your whole life is
dedicated to caring for patients, putting in long hours,
calling patients at night.*

- *Outside influences make it hard. The recertification, the
exams, seeing your income decrease and expenses go up.
Sixty percent of our income is now expenses.*

- *There is something that has changed a bit in becoming a
doctor that I didn't have to deal with. Incredible student
loans. It is incredible impact. It is a deterrent. You could go to
Wall Street or be an attorney. You can't pay them back. It
impacts who decided to be a doctor.*

- *We are used as pawns in a system. No one cares about
the doctors.*

- *They have been infantilized and taught that they shouldn't have to pay. Yet for cigarettes, the plumber, smart phone, car mechanic, they pay. Their health is the most important. And they don't expect the plumber to file with health insurance. You pay your bill. They present it to you and you pay. People are incensed at the end of a visit when they are presented with a bill. Do a surgery, save a kid's life. They take the money from the insurance company and keep it.*

- *It's hopeless. No hope in that we are looked on by people, government and agencies as the bad person.*

- *The whole training and time put in is certainly a lot of work compared to the financial rewards. It's a frustrating thing. People are looking at me like I am wealthy. I am comfortable and I am not hurting or starving. But most of my friends in business or law school are making a whole lot more money than I am. I find it frustrating at people looking at me like I am some rich guy.*

* And then there is the ever-looming threat of lawsuits.

- *I felt violated.*

- *Fear of malpractice has changed everything. When I first started in 1954, it never occurred to us that we would be sued. We never thought about it or that we would have to protect ourselves by doing an extraordinary number of tests or consultations.*

* How can we possibly see this as a tenable situation? How can this be right? How can we expect doctors to work at such a high and intense level and take care of us under these circumstances? It is absolutely amazing to me that these men and women, with this kind of pressure and with diminishing rewards, continue to function with such dedication. I don't think that I could do it. We need to stop pretending that highly trained, overworked, and underappreciated professionals will be able to continue, or will want to continue, to take care of us under these circumstances. We have a frightening and worsening doctor shortage, and the current adverse situations revealed in this book make practicing medicine very difficult.

- *Human nature and insurance companies are against us.*

- *There was a social pact in place: We provided care and we had a comfortable life. That pact was broken. The deal was broken. So now there is a new generation with a new attitude: We will provide care when we want to provide care-9-5 and no weekends.*

- *Duty hour restrictions are just for trainees. So there is more stress on the supervising MDs. There is no give in the system. We work long hours and are on call. Stressful. The other concern as a program director: Will the patients be ready when they get out there? They are restricted and do more shift work — a more difficult transition to the practice paradigm.*

- *Lots of physician burnout. The insurance companies seem to be the only ones making any money. The status of our current health is declining, not improving.*

* These powerful quotes summarize the gravity and urgency of our healthcare crisis.

* In addition to being in practice as a psychologist, I write. This is what I do. Writing this book was upsetting. Sometimes when I left the doctors after their interview, I felt physically sick or depressed. At one point, while actually writing the book, I had writer's block. I just couldn't make it happen. I was anxious and fidgety and wasted some time. This is very unusual for me. I may get a little stuck temporarily, or need to do more research, or consult with an editor or an expert, but then I move on. Not so this time, as I was finishing writing this book. I finally realized after a day or so, that what I was writing about was so upsetting and frightening, I had inadvertently allowed it to paralyze my brain.

I talked to one of my own doctors about it. I had kept her posted on the progress of this book, so this was an update. I said, "But I don't have to worry about any of this stuff, right? Because I have you." She leaned forward and said, "I will always take care of you. Finish the book." I also spoke to my insurance broker, who went into insurance when it was an honorable profession and who is appalled at the current crisis. He said, "You need to disassociate yourself from what you are writing. You are covered. Finish the book."

After talking with these two people, I was finally able to finish the book. I had to force myself to sit down and do it. I wanted to stick my head in the sand or run away. But I have a responsibility to my doctor interviewees who so generously shared with me their time and thoughts, and that motivated me to go on and finish the book.

Our healthcare crisis is but one symptom of the disturbing state of our society. It is a particularly disturbing one because it is so obviously self-destructive. Without our health, we have nothing. What has happened to our Great Society? We have become, as stated in the book with the same title, The Culture of Narcissism. Although it began much earlier, the disorganization and cultural revolt of the1960s and the self absorption and cultural upheaval of the following decades steered us away from focusing on the common good. Watergate, the Vietnam War, several assassinations (JFK, RFK, Malcolm X, MLK) all produced further societal unrest and stress. Since then, the OKC bombing, 9/11, multiple wars, another stock market crash, and the never-ending stream of interpersonal violence, have perpetuated this instability and uncertainty. In our panic and despair, we have lost sight of the fact that looking out for and caring about each other, rather than an impersonal and "wired" society, is best for each and every one of us, both individually and collectively.

The disintegration of neighborhoods and evaporation of a sense of community leaves us disconnected from each other in the truest sense, with grave consequences to our mental and physical health. We are isolated, insular and deficient in a sense of personal responsibility. Our entire well-being, and that of our nation and greater world suffers as a result. The middle class has contracted and the working poor have been hit hard by the loss of jobs through outsourcing and other job reduction policies and events. A sense of entitlement pervades our society, fueled by anger at those who use our resources, but do not work, pay taxes, or make any other substantive contribution to our society.

As part of the Great Society, Medicaid and Medicare were born. They may have been well intentioned. It is to everyone's advantage in terms of well-being, disease prevention, and finances to have healthcare for all citizens. However, my doctor interviewees see these programs as the genesis of the disintegration of our healthcare system. They placed onerous restrictions on our doctors and hospitals and spawned a sense of entitlement and reduction of personal responsibility both for care and finances.

The subsequent attempts to achieve universal healthcare, right through the Affordable Care Act, may have inched towards a desirable public policy philosophy, but have not yet reached the stated goal due to partisan politics, multiple competing constituencies, shocking greed and callousness on the part of the insurance companies, and the frank complexity of constructing a reasonable, functioning, healthcare system where all parties assume some responsibility for making it work. Comprehensive, but understandable, histories of health insurance are presented by Paul Starr and Thomas W. Loker. They are helpful in understanding the context of today's healthcare crisis.

The purpose of health insurance is to cover, reimburse, or "insure," reasonable health care costs. But through various loopholes and perhaps unintended legislative oversights or blunders, never mind the difficulties in regulating them, the health insurance industry has become a rigid benefit denying behemoth gatekeeper. A grim reaper, if you will.

As the doctor interviewees clearly and repeatedly stated, the entire healthcare system needs to change and be totally re-conceptualized and rebuilt. Financial incentives that deprive people of healthcare need to be replaced by incentives to provide people with adequate and competent care. We need tort reform, so that doctors can perform their jobs without the Damocles' sword of lawsuits hanging over their heads. We need more doctors as we have a terrifying shortage looming. In terms of the uninsured but responsible or impoverished citizens and those who are by nature of disability or illness unable to care for themselves, we need a viable plan. Perhaps we should consider returning to the days when our university medical schools provided quality healthcare for them. In return, as responsible citizens, they paid their debt to society by helping to educate our doctors in training. We need architects of the new healthcare system who understand and appreciate the complexities and hard work involved in being a doctor and providing healthcare everyday — 24/7 — on the ground. We need to address and remedy the problem of "medical tourists" and those who refuse to pay for healthcare. This is an unsustainable part of the healthcare crisis.

This book was written out of frustration, anger, and despair. I thoroughly enjoyed the time spent with each and every one of my doctor interviewees; although, at times, what they told me added to my frustration, anger, and despair. How could we possibly have allowed this situation to happen? How can we treat these people on whom our very lives depend with such disrespect?

But I also wrote this book out of the hope that armed with accurate information from our doctors who live it every day and from enough people who care and are willing to speak up and take action, we can salvage and rebuild our healthcare system before it is too late. I was in the right place, at the right time, with the right skills, with the right connections to write this book. Under those circumstances, I am constitutionally incapable of sitting still, being quiet, and doing nothing. It is not my nature.

We can't save the people who have suffered or died because the healthcare system has failed them. It is too late. We can never repay, financially or otherwise, our doctors who have sacrificed way beyond the call of duty. The system has fallen apart, now in shambles, all around them. But it is my hope that we can, in fact we must, do better at providing healthcare than what we have been doing. We have to stop pretending that we can't do any better, because we can: "Never doubt that a small group of thoughtful committed citizens can change the world; indeed, it's the only thing that ever has." (Margaret Mead).

We need to return to respecting our doctors. Our health and our very lives depend upon it. Of course there are incompetent doctors. We read about horrific examples from time to time in the press. However, if my experience with interviewing these 50 doctors has any validity, which I believe that it does, most of our doctors are good, caring, competent, well-intentioned professionals. Not perfect, mind you, because no one is perfect. We need to go back to letting them take care of us and take personal responsibility in helping them to do so. That is what they went into medicine to do. And this is what we all need from them. As one of the doctor interviewees said so poignantly, "I don't want to worry about money. I just want to be a doctor."

As I said at the beginning of this book, I wrote it for three reasons:

1. Out of incredible gratitude to my own doctors.

2. To demonstrate utmost respect for my doctor colleagues and to highlight the outrage and frustration at the disrespectful manner in which doctors are treated.

3. To educate the public and our legislators about the disturbing state of the healthcare crisis.

I firmly believe this book has accomplished the first two goals. It is now up to you, the reader, to take this knowledge and do something positive with it. Only in that manner will my third goal be reached.

REFERENCES FROM THE TEXT AND FOR FURTHER READING

Alexander, J. A., Hearld, L. R., Mittler, J. N. and Harvey, J. (2012), *Patient–Physician Role Relationships and Patient Activation among Individuals with Chronic Illness.* Health Services Research, 47: 1201–1223. doi: 10.1111/j.1475-6773.2011.01354.x
www.http://www.aafp.org/about/policies/all/mental-services.html

American Psychological Association (undated). *Psychology in Primary Care.*
www.http://www.apa.org/about/gr/issues/health-care/primary-care.aspx

Block L, Habicht R, Wu AW, Desai SV, Wang K, Silva KN, Niessen T, Oliver N, Feldman L. J Gen Intern Med. (2013) *In the wake of the 2003 and 2011 duty hours regulations, how do internal medicine interns spend their time?* Aug, 28 (8):1042-7. doi: 10.1007/s11606-013-2376-6.

Bultman, D.C. and Svarstad, B.L. (2000). *Patient Education and Counseling,* May, 40(2):173-85. *Effects of physician communication style on client medication beliefs and adherence with antidepressant treatment.*
www.http://www.ncbi.nlm.nih.gov/pubmed/10771371

Centers for Disease Control: *Workplace Health Promotion*
http://www.cdc.gov/workplacehealthpromotion/implementation/topics/depression.html

Consumer Attitudes toward Family / Primary Care Physicians and the U.S. Healthcare
System www.http://www.physiciansfoundation.org/uploads/default/Physicians_Foundation_Consumer_Omnibus_Survey.pdf

David, J.E. (2013). *Who's smiling through Obamacare blunder? Insurers, of course.*
www.http://www.cnbc.com/2013/11/15/whos-winning-obamacare-debate-publicy-traded-health-care-stocks.html

Eastwood, B. (2014). *Top health insurance CEO pay exceeds $10 million in 2014 Heads of Aetna, Anthem, Cigna, Humana, UnitedHealth earn top dollars*
www.http://www.fiercehealthpayer.com/story/top-health-insurance-ceo-pay-exceeds-10-million-2014/2015-04-10

Edwards, Haley Sweetland (March 7, 2016). *You could get hit with a surprise medical bill.*
http://time.com/4246845/health-care-insurance-suprise-medical-bill/?xid=homepage

Ehley, B. (2015). *Obamacare Gap Traps Millions With Coverage Who Can't Afford Care*
http://www.thefiscaltimes.com/2015/06/10/Obamacare-Gap-Traps-Millions-Coverage-Who-Can-t-Afford-Care

Forbes Magazine (February 21, 2016). *ACA savings: Paying doctors and hospitals bonuses to deny care to patients.*
http://www.forbes.com/sites/theapothecary/2016/02/21/aca-savings-paying-doctors-and-hospitals-bonuses-to-deny-care-to-patients/#493d07d72064

Matthews, A.W. (May 29,2015).
http://pnhp.org/blog/2015/05/29/is-blue-cross-blue-shield-an-illegal-cartel/

McCoughey, B. (2015). *ObamaCare's latest victims: 100,000 New Yorkers and taxpayers everywhere*
www.http://nypost.com/2015/09/29/obamacares-latest-victims-100000-new-yorkers-and-taxpayers-everywhere/

Minardo, J, Rothbaum, P.A., Axelbank, J. & Helfman, B. (2013). *NJPA Harnessing the Power of the Insurance Complaint Registry: Putting our data to work!* New Jersey Psychologist, 26-32. Also see www.drpeggyrothbaum.com (under "writer")

National Institute of Mental Health (undated) *Borderline Personality Disorder.*
www.http://www.nimh.nih.gov/health/topics/borderline-personality-disorder/index.shtml

NPR, The Robert Wood Johnson Foundation, Harvard T.H. Chan School of Public Health. (February, 2016). *Patients' Perspectives on Health Care in the United States.* PatientPerspectives.pdf

Healthcare from the patient perspective: The Role of the Art of Medicine in a Digital World. (2012)
Nuance.com
www.http://www.nuance.com/groups/healthcare/@webnus/documents/collateral/nc_031636.pdf

Perr, J. (2013). *Health insurers' stocks, earnings surge.*
http://www.dailykos.com/story/2013/10/29/1251599/-Health-insurers-stocks-earnings-surge#

Porter, S. (2015)
Significant Primary Care, Overall Physician Shortage Predicted by 2025.
http://www.aafp.org/news/practice-professional-issues/20150303aamcwkforce.html

Rothbaum, P.A. (March 27, 2013).
The pill is more bitter than you think.
http://www.thealternativepress.com/articles/the-pill-is-more-bitter-than-you-think
Also see www.drpeggyrothbaum.com (under "writer")

http://drpeggyrothbaum.com/blog/
I have been talking with your doctor.

Strain, L (June 17, 2015).
http://www.wsj.com/articles/antitrust-lawsuits-target-blue-cross-and-blue-shield-1432750106

U.S. News World Report (2015).
Which medical school graduates have the most debt?
www.http://grad-schools.usnews.rankingsandreviews.com/best-graduate-schools/top-medical-schools/debt-rankings

U.S. News World Report (2015).
www.http://www.usnews.com/education/best-graduate-schools/the-short-list-grad-school/articles/2015/05/19/10-medical-schools-where-students-pay-a-high-price

Whitman, E. (2015). *Rising Costs of Medical Care, Health Insurance: Median Pay For CEOs In Health Care Companies Higher Than Any Other Industry, Analysis Finds* www.http://www.ibtimes.com/rising-costs-medical-care-health-insurance-median-pay-ceos-health-care-companies-1938699

Winning, A. M., Glymour, M, McCormick, M.C. , Gilsanz, P., and Laura D. Kubzansky, L.D. 2015; 66(14):1577-1586. doi:10.1016/j.jacc.2015.08.021. *Psychological Distress Across the Life Course and Cardiometabolic Risk* (2015). Journal of the American College of Cardiology.

Witters, D., Lui, D, and Agrawal, S. (2013) http://www.cdc.gov/workplacehealthpromotion/implementation/topics/depression.html based on Gallup http://www.well-beingindex.com/

Below is a list of books to learn more about the everyday life of a doctor. Most of these books were written before the healthcare crisis became as severe as it is today. So they are a good way to understand how hard it is to train and be a doctor, even under better circumstances.

Beohm, F.H. (2001). *Doctors Cry Too.* Carlsbad, CA: Hay House, Inc.

Chen, P (2007). *Final Exam: A Surgeon's Reflections on Mortality.* New York: Knopf.

Caravella, P. (2000). *The art of being a patient.* 1st books.

Gingerich, S. (2001). *Body of Knowledge: One semester of gross anatomy: The gateway to becoming a doctor.* New York: Scribner

Groopman, J. (2007). *How Doctors Think.* New York: Houghton Mifflin Company.

Gwande, A. (2002). *Complications: A Surgeon's Notes on an Imperfect Science,* New York: Metropolitan Books.

Hilfiker, D. (1998). *Healing the Wounds: A physician looks at his work.* Omaha, Nebraska: Creighton University Press.

Klass, P (1987). *A Not Entirely Benign Procedure: Four years as a medical student.* New York: Penguin Group.

Korsch, B.M. and Harding, C. (1997). *The intelligent guide to the doctor-patient relationship.* New York: Oxford University Press.

Marion, R. (1989). *The Intern Blues: The private ordeals of three young doctors.* New York: William Morrow and Company.

Miller, C.A. (2004). *The Making of a Surgeon in the 21st Century.* Nevada City, Nevada: Blue Dolphin Press.

Ofri, D. (2013) *What Doctors Feel: How emotions affect the practice of medicine.* Boston: Beacon Press.

Pories, S., Jain, S.H., and Harper, G. (2006). *The Soul of a Doctor: Harvard medical students face life and death.* New York, Workman Press.

Rothman, E.L. (1999) *White Coat: Becoming a doctor at Harvard Medical School.* New York: HarperCollins.

Shapiro, D. (2003). *Delivering Doctor Amelia.* (2004). New York: Vintage Press.

Transue, E.R. (2004). *On Call: A Doctor's Days and Nights in Residency,* New York: St. Martin's Press.

Verghese, A. (1994). *My Own Country: A doctor's story.* New York: Vintage Books.

Watts, D. (2005). *Bedside Manners,* New York: Harmony

Books about the state of our society
Dunkelman, M.C. (2014).
The Vanishing Neighbor: The transformation of American community. New York: W.W. Norton and Company.

Herbert, B. (2014). *Losing Our Way: An intimate portrait of a troubled America.* New York, Doubleday.

Lasch, C. (1979). *The Culture of Narcissism.* New York: W.W. Norton and Company.

Putnam, R.D. (2000). *Bowling Alone: The Collapse and Revival of American Community.* New York: Simon and Schuster.

Putnam, R.D. (2015). *Our Kids: The American dream in crisis.* New York: Simon and Schuster.

Roberts, P. (2014). *The Impulse Society.* New York: Bloomsbury Publishing USA.

About healthcare
Loker, T.W. (2012). *The History and Evolution of Healthcare in America: The Untold back story of where we've been, where we are, and why healthcare needs reform.* Bloomington, IN: iUniverse.

Starr, P. (2013). *Remedy and Reflection: The peculiar American struggle over health care reform.* New Haven: Yale University Press.

Appendix 1
Interview Questions

All questions copyrighted 2012, 2013, 2014, 2015, and 2016
by Peggy A. Rothbaum, Ph. D.

Practicing Medicine

What advanced degree(s) do you hold?

Are you still practicing medicine, or are you retired?
P practicing   R retired

If still practicing, how many years have you been
in practice?

How many years have you been retired?

What is/are your specialty/ties?

Why did you leave practice, you are no longer practicing?

Being a Doctor

Why did you become a doctor?

What are the most desirable qualities of a doctor?
What are the necessary skills and abilities?

Please tell me about a typical day or week for you

What are your greatest strengths as a doctor?

What was your greatest joy in your career as a doctor?

What was your proudest moment as a doctor?

What did you do as a doctor that really made
a difference?

What was your lowest point in your career as a doctor?

What was your most difficult experience or hardest day as a doctor?

What was your biggest disappointment as a doctor?

What was your biggest stress as a doctor?
   How did you handle it?
   How did you feel about it?
   What does the job entail?

Why is it so hard to be a doctor?
What does the public need to understand?

How did you balance your personal life with being a doctor?

How did you/do you handle all of the feelings that go along with being a doctor?

What did you need that you didn't have?

THE PATIENTS

What is it/was it like working with patients?

Please tell me your thoughts on the doctor-patient relationship. Does it matter? If so, why?

Please tell me about your most difficult patient/s?

What made this/these pateints so difficult?

How did you handle it?

How did you feel at the time?
   Looking back on it?

In general, did patients get more or less difficult, or stay the same, over the years?

Please describe your favorite patient/s.
    Why?

Did you have any traumatized patients?
    What kind of trauma?

Did you have any patients with Borderline Personality Disorder?
    Describe please.

What role does mental health play in healthcare?

Do you think that the patients understand how hard it is to be a doctor
    Does the general public?

Please explain to me the complexity of being a doctor.
    Why is this so hard for patients and the general public to understand?

Is there anything that you have not been able to forget?
    Anyone?

Being a Doctor Now

Is being a doctor different now than it was when you first started?
    If so, why?
    If so, how?
    If so, when?

Has practice changed?
    If so, why?
    If so, how?
    If so, when?

If you had it to do all over again, would you become a doctor?
   Why?
   Why not?

Is training to be a doctor different now?
   If so, how?

Are the younger doctors different now?
   If so, how?

Do they have anything that you didn't have?

Are they missing something that you had?

What is their biggest source of stress?

What would you like to tell them?

What do they need that they don't have?

What needs to change?

How can this be accomplished?

What is/are the biggest unresolved issue(s) in medicine?

Why is this so hard to understand?

THE HEALTHCARE CRISIS

What is the current state of healthcare?

How would you summarize the healthcare crisis?

Is this different than it used to be?
If so, how?
When did you first notice?
What is wrong with it?
How and when did this happen?
How does this affect you as a doctor?
How does it affect your patients?
How does it affect the doctor-patient relationship?

Has the insurance situation changed being a doctor?
If so, how?

Why are the patients so reluctant to understand
the problem?

Why are they so angry about it?

What are some solutions to the healthcare crisis?
What has to change?
How can this happen?

Would you share some of your feelings about it all?

What has been lost?

Can we get it back?
How?

Appendix 2
Chapter Indexes

Index Chapter 2

Why did you become a doctor?

It was a way to combine science with interacting with people.

What are the most desirable qualities of a doctor?
What are the necessary skills and abilities?

Caring, and being able to show it.

Caring combined with clinical skills.

Being able to juggle the demanding requirements.

Persistence and not giving up.

Need to recognize limits in their own abilities.

Flexibility to adapt to change.

Being flexible is not enough.

Please tell me about a typical day or week for you.

24/7

I am always on.

I take my iPad with me wherever I go.

What are your greatest strengths as a doctor?

Caring.

Persistence.

Clinical skills.

WHAT WAS YOUR GREATEST JOY IN YOUR CAREER AS A DOCTOR?

Interactions with patients.

Pride in clinical accomplishments.

WHAT WAS YOUR PROUDEST MOMENT AS A DOCTOR?

Caring.

Pride in clinical accomplishments.

WHAT DID YOU DO AS A DOCTOR THAT REALLY MADE A DIFFERENCE?

Caring.

Clinical skills.

The doctor patient relationship.

WHAT WAS YOUR LOWEST POINT IN YOUR CAREER AS A DOCTOR?

Business issues, including lawsuits.

Feelings about their lives.

Patient care.

WHAT WAS YOUR MOST DIFFICULT EXPERIENCE OR HARDEST DAY AS A DOCTOR?

Business and insurance issues.

Clinical work load.

Patient deaths.

Very sick patients.

Giving patients bad news.

WHAT WAS YOUR BIGGEST DISAPPOINTMENT AS
A DOCTOR?

Business and insurance issues.

Patient relationships.

Negative patient behavior.

Business and practice issues.

WHAT WAS YOUR BIGGEST STRESS AS A DOCTOR?
HOW DID YOU HANDLE IT? HOW DID YOU FEEL ABOUT IT

Lawsuits.

Business and practice issues.

Patient care.

Personal issues.

WHAT DOES THE JOB ENTAIL?

Clinical skills and caring.

WHY IS IT SO HARD TO BE A DOCTOR? WHAT DOES THE
PUBLIC NEED TO UNDERSTAND?

This society accepts no mistakes.

The public and the government expect you to do the
impossible. Take care of patients flawlessly with
no money.

Because medicine is an art, not a science.

Because you are responsible for things that you
can't control.

It's not really a job, it's your life.

Because nobody appreciates the degree of stress,
thought, and time that goes into it.

Death and dying and paperwork. That we are
being bogged down by a bunch of bullshit.

**HOW DID YOU BALANCE YOUR PERSONAL LIFE WITH BEING
A DOCTOR?**

It's a constant struggle.

Give up and miss out on a lot.

Some solutions and strategies.

**HOW DID YOU/DO YOU HANDLE ALL OF THE FEELINGS THAT
GO ALONG WITH BEING A DOCTOR?**

It's a challenge.

Support.

WHAT DID YOU NEED THAT YOU DIDN'T HAVE?

No unmet needs

Unmet needs.

INDEX CHAPTER 3

WHAT IS IT/WAS IT LIKE WORKING WITH PATIENTS?

A positive experience

Clinically interesting

Some negatives

PLEASE TELL ME YOUR THOUGHTS ON THE DOCTOR-PATIENT RELATIONSHIP. DOES IT MATTER? IF SO, WHY?

It's everything. No disagreement here in these interviews.

The doctor patient relationship has changed, and not for the better.

PLEASE TELL ME ABOUT YOUR MOST DIFFICULT PATIENT/S?

Clinical difficulties

Abusive, ungrateful, manipulative, or entitled patients

Other negative patient behavior

Difficult families

Non-compliance

WHAT MADE THIS/THESE PATIENTS SO DIFFICULT?

Entitlement

HOW DID YOU HANDLE IT?

Strategies and acceptance

Educating or setting limits

Asking the patience to leave

Persistence

How did you feel at the time? Looking back on it?

In general, did patients get more or less difficult, or stay the same, over the years?

The same

More difficult

Easier

Insurance issues

Please describe your favorite patient/s. Why?

Certain age groups

Those where there is a relationship

Appreciation and the relationship

Did you have any traumatized patients? What kinds of trauma?

Many different types

Did you have any patients with Borderline Personality Disorder? Describe please.

Yes

What role does mental health play in healthcare?

A big one

Problems with insurance

Do you think that the patients understand how hard it is to be a doctor?

A vast majority of "no" responses

Some do

Dᴏᴇs ᴛʜᴇ ɢᴇɴᴇʀᴀʟ ᴘᴜʙʟɪᴄ?

A vast majority of "no" responses

Some do

Pʟᴇᴀsᴇ ᴇxᴘʟᴀɪɴ ᴛᴏ ᴍᴇ ᴛʜᴇ ᴄᴏᴍᴘʟᴇxɪᴛʏ ᴏғ ʙᴇɪɴɢ ᴀ ᴅᴏᴄᴛᴏʀ. Wʜʏ ɪs ᴛʜɪs sᴏ ʜᴀʀᴅ ғᴏʀ ᴘᴀᴛɪᴇɴᴛs ᴀɴᴅ ᴛʜᴇ ɢᴇɴᴇʀᴀʟ ᴘᴜʙʟɪᴄ ᴛᴏ ᴜɴᴅᴇʀsᴛᴀɴᴅ?

Time

Hard work

Insurance problems

Providing

 correct care

Is ᴛʜᴇʀᴇ ᴀɴʏᴛʜɪɴɢ ᴛʜᴀᴛ ʏᴏᴜ ʜᴀᴠᴇ ɴᴏᴛ ʙᴇᴇɴ ᴀʙʟᴇ ᴛᴏ ғᴏʀɢᴇᴛ? Aɴʏᴏɴᴇ?

Powerful stories

Difficult clinical situations

Is training to be a doctor different now?

Yes, It's all shiftwork. Positive clinical differences

If so, how?

Are the younger doctors different now?

Yes, they are shift workers. and They come out looking for a 9-5 job.

If so, how?

Do they have anything that you didn't have?
Are they missing something that you had?

Yes

Technology

A different work ethic

Debt

A personal life

Duty hours

No. They are still starry eyed and they are going to save the world.

What is their biggest source of stress?

Finances

Time

Clinical stresses

What would you like to tell them?

It's worth it.

Medicine is not 9-5.

The importance of humanism

WHAT DO THEY NEED THAT THEY DON'T HAVE?

Experience

Time with patients

Less financial stress

WHAT NEEDS TO CHANGE?

The basics of the healthcare system

Time with patients

HOW CAN THAT BE ACCOMPLISHED?

WHAT IS/ARE THE BIGGEST UNRESOLVED ISSUE(S) IN MEDICINE? WHY IS THIS SO HARD TO UNDERSTAND?

Payment

Insurance

Access

Tort reform

Index Chapter 5

What is the current state of healthcare?

It's a nightmare from every angle.

Abominable and it's immoral

Unstable

Frightening

How would you summarize the healthcare crisis?

Insurance problems

Entitlement

Access

Lawsuits

Is this different than it used to be? If so, how?

Insurance problems

Denial of care

When did you first notice?

Over time

What is wrong with it?

People are making decisions that they are not trained to make. They are not physicians.

There is no care of the patients, it's all about money.

How and why did this happen?

Greed

Entitlement

Insurance problems

HOW DOES THIS AFFECT YOU AS A DOCTOR?

Patient care

Insurance problems

HOW DOES IT AFFECT THE PATIENTS?

Patient care

Accessibility

HOW DOES IT AFFECT THE DOCTOR-PATIENT RELATIONSHIP?

Almost destroys it. Less time Entitlement

HAS THE INSURANCE SITUATION CHANGED BEING A DOCTOR? IF SO, HOW?

Finances

Patient care

The insurance companies do not want patients to live.

They make more money if the patients die.

WHY ARE THE PATIENTS SO RELUCTANT TO UNDERSTAND THE PROBLEM?

Unrealistic expectations

Entitlement

They blame the doctors

Insurance problems

It's complicated.

WHY ARE THEY SO ANGRY ABOUT IT?

They feel powerless and helpless.

Entitlement

They don't understand.

**WHAT ARE SOME SOLUTIONS TO THE HEALTHCARE CRISIS?
WHAT HAS TO CHANGE? HOW CAN THIS HAPPEN?**

Insurance and malpractice reform

Provide better care

WOULD YOU SHARE SOME OF YOUR FEELINGS ABOUT IT ALL?

Insurance

Quality of care

Malpractice reform

Administrative costs

WHAT HAS BEEN LOST?

Patient care

The doctor-patient relationship

Respect for doctors

Insurance problems

Malpractice

CAN WE GET IT BACK? HOW?

There is not a lot of optimism from the doctor interviewees
in answer to this question.

CPSIA information can be obtained
at www.ICGtesting.com
Printed in the USA
LVHW01*2204200817
545701LV00012B/321/P